LEAN & GREEN DIET

Table Of Contents

Introduction

Optavia diet enhances weight loss through branded products known as "Fuelings" while the homemade entrées are referred to as the "Lean and Green" meals. The Fuelings are made up of over 60 items, specifically low in carbs (carbohydrates) but high in probiotic cultures and protein. The fuelings ultimately contain friendly bacteria that can help boost gut health. They include cookies, bars, puddings, shakes, soups, cereals, and pasta.

Looking at the listed foods, you might think they are relatively high in carbs, which is understandable, but the Fuelings are composed so that they are lower in sugar and carbs than the traditional versions of similar foods. The company does this by using small-portion sizes and sugar substitutes. Many of the Fuelings are packed with soy protein isolate and whey protein powder in furtherance. Those who are interested in the Optavia diet plan but are not interested in cooking or have no chance for it are provided with pre-made, low-carb meals. These meals are referred to as "Flavors of Home," and they can sufficiently replace the Lean and Green Meals.

The company explicitly states that by working with its team of coaches and following the Optavia diet as required, you will achieve a "lifelong transformation, one healthy habit at a time."

Therefore, to record success with this diet plan, you have to stick to the Fuelings supplemented by veggie, meat, and healthy fat entrée daily; you will be full and nourished. Although you will be consuming low calories, you will not be losing a lot of muscle since you will be feeding on lots of fiber, protein, and other vital nutrients. Your calories as an adult will not exceed 800–1,000. You can lose 12 pounds in 12 weeks if you follow the 5&1 Optimal Weight Plan option.

Since you will curb your carb intake while on this diet plan, you will naturally shed fat because the carb is the primary source of energy, therefore, if it is not readily available, the body finds a fat alternative, which implies that the body will have to break down your fats for energy and keep burning fat.

Finally, with this book, you will determine if the Optavia diet program is a weight loss program convenient for you before you get started.

"I'm on a diet. I can't come for the weekend!" Punctually said Martha, a friend I have known since adolescence. She was always struggling with weight; she never saw herself right, and when we went out with the others, she had constant difficulties in choosing fashionable clothes like all of us. In reality, he didn't have that many kg in excess...

maybe 5–6...? But this caused her low self-esteem and insecurity in any social context. After 27 years of diets, she got married and had a beautiful baby. Martha, during pregnancy, gained 30 kilograms! So that suffering resurfaces for her appearance, for the joint pains that lead her not to sleep at night, lethargy, and that sense of discomfort with her husband who saw her only with those XXL clothes. She was tired of diets that started on Monday and stopped for the weekend. She needed a fast, definitive, serious path, but above all, a support that would help her manage meals because now, with a family, she couldn't stop cooking and isolate herself.

So she knew the Optavia Diet, a low-carb path with a high-protein content, and is immediately struck because it was based on a choice of over 60 healthy and fast solutions, including shakes, bars, soups, biscuits, salty snacks ... high content protein, with probiotics and prebiotics to promote correct absorption of nutrients and good digestion. In this way, she no longer had to waste time and money in supermarkets, looking for refined and unavailable ingredients!! She could choose between 3 different routes that would bring her to a healthy weight. Martha chose the strongest and fastest 5&1, moving on to 4&2&1 and then to 3&3. It is a path that is not based only on substitute meals but also on cooked meals, precisely to not become slaves to a product and learn to eat while losing weight healthily, not affecting lean mass. After a short time, her appearance began to change, not only for the loss of weight and size, but
for that radiant light on her face, different energy, and for the first time I saw her sitting at the table serene, without having to give up her social life. This book is for all those women who often step aside, at the expense of their happiness, but who deserve a new chance.

Martha finally found her solution with the Optavia diet, eliminating those 30 kgs in a few months and entering the size 40 she had always sought. To date, after two years, it has never started again, dispelling the myth that by following low-calorie routes, one gains weight quickly. First of all, because with this diet you eat 6 times a day and the kg you recover is determined exclusively by the incorrect lifestyle, you are applying at that moment and not by the previous one. This book also serves as mental support on approaching a definitive path of transformation and is perhaps my favorite part because it is essential to keep in mind why you started and where you want to go. I believe that each of us deserves to feel better, feel full of energy, and not underestimate ourselves as a woman!!

And since we women like to share our secrets, here you can find many: on how not to finally give up on social life, how to organize yourself with meals, how to meet the needs of the whole family, how to find yourself without guilt and many healthy, practical and tasty recipes that will lead you to be satisfied even in the kitchen, regaining your physical shape, and without having to count calories anymore! You will have a list of foods to prefer and avoid that you can always carry with you and some practical tricks on smart shopping! We will start with the first action: cleaning the kitchen pantries of all those pre-packaged foods, which intoxicate us, make room for healthy foods, and combine them in a conscious, stimulating, and fun way! And then, let's face it: the healthier you eat, the more your body will ask for healthy things! Enjoy this book and your wellness journey with the Optavia diet!

CHAPTER 1:
Optavia Diet's Mindset

A can't see it on the scale. Just think of it as one big step closer, even if it feels like a small step. I would advise you not to weigh yourself every day as this may put you off, and any progress might seem like it's happening syouknow,youwillnotloseweightovernight,soit'sgoodtokeepamindset thateverydaycountsevenifyou
too slow. Stick to once a week at the same time in the mornings. If you do weigh yourself at different times, do not be alarmed if you seem to put on weight, as it can and will fluctuate during the day and throughout the week. This is because of the things you consume and how your body handles them.

You can also look at it as a game or challenge to become fun rather than something you hate. The best way to do this is to find another person to share your progress with. This can be friends or family or even people you don't know and sometimes a group. Because you have the same goals as other people out there, you may even make some new friends.

You can make certain meals feel like a treat even though they are nowhere near as bad as some of your usual eating habits, but you can still fill that desire. Moderation and better choices come into play here, so don't order the burger and fries. Have a chicken salad instead.

Every time you look in the fridge and spot something you really shouldn't be eating, think of that food in the future and not the present. It may taste nice when you eat it, but you will feel guilty afterward, and a few days after that, the scale may not show the progress you wanted it to show, so just think ahead of time before making any decision when making food choices.

People may make fun of you for choosing to exercise and diet. They may not believe in you for whatever reason. This may be because they could not imagine themselves changing their lifestyle in such a way, so in their eyes, you must also fail at it. Shrug it off and continue as usual, and you will be the one laughing when you reach your goals. It's not an issue what other people think as it's your actions that dictate your outcome. To achieve this, you need to let go of all your fears that could make it harder for you and concentrate on the result.

Sometimes when you are doing well, you may treat yourself a little too much, and then it backfires, and you end up doing more damage to your progress than you could have imagined. Instead of treating yourself to something bad to eat, you could challenge yourself to have something healthy in place of that treat and then feel twice as good later. Self-satisfaction is the biggest reward. Remember, it's still excellent to treat yourself every now and again to avoid binging. Have a cheat meal or a cheat day but fit it into your daily calorie limit.

Sticking to Good Habits

Most people want to be the best person they can be. They want to live healthy, well-rounded lives that satisfy them. They usually all know what they SHOULD be doing on a day-to-day basis to achieve this life they desire. So why is it so hard to stick to good habits? Why do we get motivated for short periods only to fall back into bad habits a short time later?

Have you ever resolved to add a healthy habit to your life? Lose 20 pounds? Eat healthier? Increase the amount of weight you can lift? Chances are, if you are like most, you started those practices with the best intentions, only to get sidetracked somewhere along the way, and they never became habits. Why does that happen so consistently to so many of us? The answer is that we try to make changes in the wrong way. In attempting to change the wrong way, there is little possibility for something to become a lasting change. This book will show you a better strategy to finally make long term changes in your life successfully.

Do's & Don'ts of the Optavia Diet

The Optavia diet plan has some guidelines—especially in food consumption—that must be adhered to if you wish to record a diet plan successfully.

Recommended Foods to Eat

The foods you are liable to eat while on the 5&1 plan are the 5 Optavia Fuelings and 1 Lean and Green meal daily.

The meals consist mainly of healthy fats, lean protein, and low-carb vegetables, and there is a recommendation for only two servings of fatty fish every week. Some beverages and low-carb condiments are also allowed in small proportions.

The Foods that Are allowed for the Lean and Green Meals

- **Fish and Shellfish:** Trout, tuna, halibut, salmon, crab, scallops, lobster, and shrimp
- **Meat:** Lean beef, lamb, chicken, game meats, turkey, tenderloin or pork chop, and ground meat (must be 85% lean at least)
- **Vegetable Oils:** Walnut, flaxseed, olive oil, and canola
- **Eggs:** Whole Eggs, egg beaters, and egg whites

- **Additional Healthy Fats:** Reduced-fat margarine, walnuts, pistachios, almonds, avocado, olives, and low carb salad dressings
- **Soy Products:** Tofu
- **Sugar-free Beverages:** Unsweetened almond milk, coffee, tea, and water
- **Sugar-free Snacks:** Gelatin, mints, popsicles, and gum
- **Low-Carb Vegetables:** Celery, mushrooms, cauliflower, zucchini, peppers, jicama, spinach, cucumbers, cabbage, eggplant, broccoli, spaghetti squash, and collard greens
- **Seasonings and Condiments:** Lemon juice, yellow mustard, salsa, zero-calorie sweeteners, barbecue sauce, cocktail sauce, dried herbs, salt, spices, lime juice, soy sauce, sugar-free syrup, and ½ teaspoons only of ketchup

Summary: The Optavia 5&1 plan's homemade meals consist mainly of low-carb veggies, lean proteins, and a few healthy fats. It allows only low-carb beverages like unsweetened almond milk, water, tea, and coffee.

Foods That Are Not Allowed

Apart from the carbs contained in the pre-packaged Optavia fuelings, most carb-containing beverages and foods are not allowed while you are on the 5&1 plan. Some fats are also banned as well as all fried foods.

Below are the foods you must avoid, except if they are included in your Fuelings:

- **Refined Grains:** Pasta, pancakes, crackers, cookies, pastries, white bread, biscuits, flour tortillas, white rice, and cakes
- **Fried Foods:** Fish, vegetables, shellfish, meats, and sweets like pastries
- **Whole Fat Dairy:** Cheese, milk, and yogurt
- **Certain Fats:** Coconut oil, butter, and solid shortening
- **Sugar-Sweetened Beverages:** fruit juice, soda, energy drinks, sports drinks, and sweet tea
- **Alcohol:** All varieties

The foods below are banned while on the 5&1 plan but are added to the 6-week transition phase and with no restriction during the 3&3 plan:

- **Fruits:** All fresh fruits
- **Whole Grains:** High-fibre breakfast cereal, whole grain bread, whole-wheat pasta, and brown rice
- **Starch Vegetables:** Corn, white potatoes, sweet potatoes, and peas
- **Low-Fat or Fat-Free Dairy:** Milk, yogurt, and cheese
- **Legumes:** Beans, peas, lentils, and soybeans

Note that during the 6-week transition phase, and while on the 3&3 plan, you are advised to eat more berries if you must take fruits as they contain lower carbs.

Fundamentals of Optavia Diet

Optavia is a fast weight reduction or maintenance method that prescribes a combination of bought, refined foods labeled "Fueling" and "Lean and Green" home-made meals. There's no carbohydrates or calories counting. Instead,

as part of six-or-so small meals every day, members apply water to a powdered meal or unwrap a cookie.

The purpose of introducing Fuelings is to curb the cravings and a nutritiously balanced meal to keep the dieter satiated.

Based on the requirements of a person, there are three different low-calorie strategies to choose from.

1. The 5&1 plan requires 5 Optavia Fuelings and 1 Lean and Green meal, and it consists of vegetables and proteins (for example, broccoli and chicken), which are included in the 5&1 Program.
2. The 4&2&1 strategy requires 4 Fuelings, 2 Lean and Green meals, and 1 light snack (like a slice of fruit) for a bit more variety.
3. The 3&3 package, which involves 3 Fuelings and 3 Lean and Green products, for those participating in weight management.

Optavia also presents trainers with instructions to help you develop their "Habits of Health." The strategy also advises performing approximately 30 minutes of exercise with mild intensity every day and consuming more than 64 ounces of water daily.

This Optavia diet is meant to help individuals reduce weight and obesity by portion-controlled snacks and meals by lowering carbohydrates and calories.

Understanding a Low-Carb Diet

Tbut the ones that proved to be beneficial to managing diabetes substituted the carbs with healthy fats. That way, it becomes a low-carb, high-fat diet. If you are going to cut the carbs, you need to provide your body with anhedefinitionofalow-carbdietisonethathasminimalcarbohydrates.Therearemanytypesoflow-carbdiets, alternative energy source, which is healthy fats in this case.

That means significantly minimizing or cutting out high-starch foods and carbs such as rice, pasta, processed sugary foods, foods containing flour, like white bread, while loading up your diet with high-fiber and low-glycemic-index foods such as vegetables, healthy fats, and proteins to a lesser extent.

Managing your weight with a low-carb diet is a healthy way to lose weight and promote your overall health. It converts your body from being a sugar-burning machine into a fat-burning machine. However, note that there is a transition period of about 7 to 14 days before your body wholly and successfully switches from burning sugars to burning fats. During this transition period, your body will suffer from mild changes due to carbs deprivation (remember, it still depends on carbs during the transition period).

Problems with a Low-Carb Diet

You will also face initial fatigue from the shift in your diet and lower your glucose intake. If you have type 1 diabetes, you need to be very careful about making dietary habit changes. This requires modification of your insulin dose, so you need to consult your doctor before making any diet changes. The fewer carbohydrates you ingest, the less insulin you will need, and therefore, you will not need the same amount of insulin dose you used to take when you were having a regular or high-carb diet.

As your body transitions from a high-carb state to a low-carb state, you will face some problems, but this should not discourage you. Here is a list of issues that you may face in the short transition period when you initially start a low-carb diet:

You may start to feel lightheaded or dizzy, get headaches or feel fatigued, but this will quickly go away within a few days as your body starts to adapt to using fats for energy instead of sugars. If this problem persists or affects your normal daily functions, stop the low-carb diet immediately, and consult your doctor.

You may find yourself having problems with retaining water, as the carbohydrates help in water retention. When you decrease your carb intake, you will start to shed more water than your body typically loses. Loss of water is often accompanied by loss of salt; this may lead you to feel cramps or experience rapid heartbeats. You may also feel your pressure drop due to the loss of water. You can compensate by drinking lots of water and adding minerals to it. These changes are only temporary and should subside after some time; however, if you remain tired, dizzy, or sleepy, consult your doctor immediately.

Aren't Fats Unhealthy?

We mentioned that it is important to include fat in the replacement of the decreased carb intake. This raises the question, "aren't fats unhealthy?" It is a misconception to assume that fats are unhealthy. They are an essential component in our body. Your body needs fats to synthesize many hormones—and this goes into the composition of our cell membrane. Fats are also heat-insulators, preserving your body's heat. They also lie around your vital organs, such as the kidney, protecting it from trauma. A moderate amount of fat is necessary for a healthy body. However, the problem with fats occurs when they exceed the normal range.

There are healthy fats and unhealthy fats. The same goes for cholesterol. There is good cholesterol and bad cholesterol. Fish, olive oil and eggs, etc., contain natural fats. However, synthetic hydrogenated fats are considered an unhealthy type.

Good cholesterol is associated with HDL (high-density lipoprotein), which is a healthy and desirable type of cholesterol, as it helps lower your lipids and improve your lipid profile. This contrasts with LDL (low-density lipoprotein), which has undesirable health effects on your body. Therefore, it is essential to distinguish between the different types of fats to know what foods to opt for and what foods to avoid. Examples of healthy fats include monounsaturated fats and polyunsaturated fats.

Examples of Monounsaturated Fats

- Avocados, olives, peanut butter, oils like sesame oil, peanut oil, canola oil, and olive oil

  Nuts like peanuts, almonds, hazelnuts, pecans, and cashews

Examples of Polyunsaturated Fats

- Sunflower seeds, sesame seeds, and pumpkin seeds
- Nuts like walnuts
- Fatty fish like salmon, tuna, mackerel, sardines, and fish oil
- Plant oils like soya bean and safflower oil
- Tofu and soya milk

Examples of unhealthy fats include trans fats and saturated fats.

Examples of Trans Fats

- All the commercially-baked cookies, doughnuts, pastries, muffins, pizza dough, etc.
- Packaged snacks such as microwave popcorn, chips, or crackers
- Hydrogenated margarine

  Fried food such as fried chicken, chicken

  nuggets, breaded fish, and French fries
- Food that contains hydrogenated
- vegetable oils

Examples of Saturated Fats

- Chicken skin
- Hydrogenated butter
- Ice cream
- Fatty meat

General Habits to Decrease Your Carb Intake

There are many ways to decrease your carb intake. Everything lies in the small habits, especially your shopping habits, as that is where it all begins. When you are shopping, avoid items like bakeries in general and pastries full of carbs. Instead, load up your shopping cart with vegetables. Did you know that you can have 20 grams of carbs by either a plateful of assorted vegetables or a slice of bread? Guess which one makes you feel fuller and which one is healthier?

Start substituting main course items with healthy alternatives. For example, you can replace rice with cauliflower by grinding it in a blender to make cauliflower rice. It is almost the same and is much healthier.

You can also replace the pastries in your shopping cart with healthy alternatives, such as meat, eggs, chicken, and foods that make you feel full while again loading your body with beneficial nutrients.

When you are shopping, avoid shopping for processed foods or candy and sweets. They are full of artificial sweeteners and sugars that will cause you to exceed the physiological recommended carb limit with just a few bites.

Instead, you can opt for fruits. They are like candy from nature; however, be careful to choose foods with a low glycemic index, such as avocados, strawberries, berries, peaches, etc. Decrease your intake of fruits that have a high glycemic index, such as bananas.

Energy drinks, sports drinks, and fizzy drinks are dangerous not only to your diet but also to your health. If you love having fluids, it is an excellent option to blend some low-glycemic fruits and make a smoothie or drink plenty of water or skimmed milk. It is much healthier in terms of managing weight and promoting your overall health to drink fruit smoothies, as they contain lots of nutrients and vitamins that are beneficial for your overall health. Sweetened tea, coffee with sugar, flavored coffee or chocolate drinks, and energy drinks are some of the worst options you can have as they are full of sugars. Instead, you can have black coffee with low-fat milk.

Snacking can be one of the subconscious ways to load up on sugars without even realizing it. All those chips, crisps, and crackers are full of artificial flavors and refined, processed sugars. A healthy option is to snack on celery or carrots. Snacking on cucumber bites with tahini sauce is a very healthy low-carb snack option full of fibers beneficial for your colon health and helps lower your cholesterol.

Meat, fish and seafood, chicken, and eggs are proteins that are good for you. Keep the meat low in fat. If you are eating poultry, trim the skin off. Moreover, it is better to go for plant-based protein as you will get more nutrients and fibers that are not present in animal products. Try to avoid fried meat or meat with high-fat cuts; for example, ribs, pork, bacon, added cheese, or deep-fried fish are all unhealthy options due to the added unhealthy fats.

Fats, oils, and sweets are some of the favorite food of many people; however, you need to be extra careful about your choice of fats from natural sources; for example, vegetables, nut seeds, and avocados are very healthy. However, try to keep to small proportions of foods that also give you Omega-3 fatty acids, such as salmon, tuna, and mackerel. Other healthy options are grape seed oil, olive oil, and plant-based oils. For healthy options, try to avoid anything that has trans-fat in it and also avoid partially-hydrogenated fats.

It can be challenging initially, but you have to skip desserts such as ice cream and any sugar-loaded food. You can keep those options as a reward on your cheat day. If you are craving a dessert, you can try dipping some low glycemic index fruits in some heavy whipping cream or cream cheese while topping it off with berries. This is a very healthy way to stay low in carbs while also gaining fat, which you need. If you absolutely must have chocolates, it is a much healthier option to go for dark chocolate; however, try not to do that often.

The Optavia diet provides convenience to people as it is a convenient meal replacement that removes the guesswork for many of its dieters. The Optavia Diet, previously known as "Medifast," was developed by Dr. William Vitale and encouraged people to eat healthy to achieve sustainable weight loss.

Under this diet regimen, dieters follow a weight loss plan, including five Fuelings a day and one Lean and Green meal. One of the popular diet plans that Optavia offers is the 5&1 plan designed for rapid weight loss. With this diet plan, users need to eat five of Optavia's Fuelings and one Lean and Green meal daily.

With the meal replacement and Lean and Green meals, this diet is perfect for people who want to lose weight and wish to transition from their old unhealthy habits to a healthier one. Thus, this is perfect for people who suffer from gout, diabetes, and people in their senior years.

Because it is a commercial diet, it has been subjected to different studies involving its efficacy. Studies have noted that people can lose weight in as little as 8 weeks; therefore, this is one of the most efficient diet regimens there is, as people can adapt and eventually embrace it as part of their lifestyles. Read on to learn about the Optavia diet.

Foods to Avoid When on Low-Carb

Beverages That Are Sweetened with Sugar

These beverages are some of the worst choices to obtain. This is because they are very high in carbs. For example, a 12-ounce can of soda has roughly 38 grams of carbs. The same applies to sweetened iced tea or sweetened lemonade as they contain about 35 grams of carbs per serving.

Trans Fats

These are fats that are made by adding hydrogen to unsaturated fatty acids to stabilize them. Examples of trans fats can be found in margarine and frozen dinners. Besides, many food companies add trans fats to the muffins and baked goods for better taste and extend their expiry date.

Trans fats do not directly affect raising your blood glucose levels; however, they increase your insulin resistance and promote the accumulation of fat.

Don't disturb your fat metabolism and decrease your good cholesterol because this has the indirect effect of losing control of your weight management.

Pasta, Rice and White Bread

All these foods are rich in carbohydrates and quickly get digested to release lots of glucose into the blood. Besides, these foods are low in nutrients and have very little fiber, so the overall nutritional value is almost insignificant. Food rich in fiber is essential for controlling weight, cholesterol levels, and blood pressure; therefore, the main bulk of your food should be dedicated to foods that are high in fiber.

Fruit-Flavored Yogurt

Simple plain yogurt is a very healthy option. On the contrary, yogurt that is fruit-flavored is entirely different. They are often made from non-fat milk, and they are loaded with carbohydrates and sugars. One serving of fruit-flavored yogurt has about 47 grams of carbohydrates in the form of sugar. Instead of choosing yogurt that is flavored and rich in sugars, opt for simple, sugar-free, whole milk yogurt, which is helpful for your gut health and helps lose weight.

Fruits to Avoid

Grapes

A single grape contains 1 gram of carbohydrates, which means if you eat 30 grapes, you are easily eating 30 grams of carbs. And you can eat the same number of berries or strawberries while having significantly less amount of carbohydrates.

Cherries

They are super delicious; that is why it is hard to stop eating them once you have started; however, they are very rich in sugars and can cause your blood sugar to spike quickly.

Pineapple

When fresh and ripe, they can have a very high glycemic index. If you must eat pineapples, try to have a small serving of about half a cup and eat it with low-fat food, for example, Greek yogurt. Don't eat canned pineapple, as they are sweetened with unhealthy sugars.

Mango

These are super delicious foods; however, one single mango has about 30 grams of carbohydrates and nearly 25 grams of sugars. A riper and softer mango will have a higher glycemic index, while a firm mango will have a relatively lower glycemic index.

Banana

It is one of those too sweet yet very delicious foods. A medium-sized banana has about the same ounces of carbohydrates, which is double of any other fruit.

If you must have a banana, try to have half a serving and refrigerate the rest of it for another time.

Dried fruits seem harmless, especially when you add them to your food; however, two tablespoons of dried raisins have a similar amount of carbohydrates as just one cup of blueberries or another small piece of another fruit. That is because the water content has dried out, and their sugars have significantly been concentrated. Remove dried fruits from your diet and add fresh ones to your diet instead.

General Guide When Choosing Food to Eat

No matter what kind of diet you are attempting to follow, it is not correct to eliminate an entire food group. While on low carb, you can try minimizing your intake of starch and sugars but don't fall prey to the mistake of eliminating starch as your body needs carbs. Instead, you must choose wisely between the various food options in each category to ensure that you ingest the best and most suitable food type from each category and avoid the ones that will worsen your condition.

The goal of controlling your food with Optavia is eating food that will not increase your blood glucose levels higher than usual. At the same time, it needs to be food that makes you feel full and keeps hunger at bay; besides, specific food categories can promote your health and provide you with nutritional elements that can help you fight off your weight increase and protect you from its complications.

Low-Starch Food

Whole grains, for example, oatmeal, quinoa, and brown rice, are preferred and healthier than white rice, white flour or processed grains, macaroni, etc.

Baked sweet potato provides a low-carb option in contrast to regular potatoes, such as French fries. Other items that are high in carbs include white bread and white flour etc. Instead, opt for whole-grain foods that have very little added sugar or none at all.

Non-Starchy Vegetables

One of the healthiest options if you have diabetes is to include a couple of servings of non-starchy vegetables per day. There is very little chance that you could go wrong with overeating non-starchy vegetables; that is because they have a deficient calorific intake.

Non-starchy vegetables are vegetables that contain a small number of carbohydrates. This is typically about 5 grams or less of carbohydrates per 100 grams of serving non-starchy vegetables.

It should be your goal throughout your day that you have at least five portions of fruit and vegetables, and out of those 5, it is best to have at least three of them that are non-starchy vegetables.

There are several reasons why non-starchy vegetables are very healthy options for low carb. The foremost reason is that they are deficient in carbs. Other causes include how non-starchy vegetables are very nutritious. They are full of vitamins and minerals as well as other critical nutrients such as phytochemicals. Besides being vegetables, they are a crucial source of dietary fiber. Dietary fiber will help you digest food properly, and it also plays an essential role in
 lowering your cholesterol levels. Overall, dietary fiber is a crucial nutrient to include in your diet.

Non-starchy vegetables are also rich in vitamins and minerals such as vitamin A, vitamin C, and vitamin K. Vitamin C helps promote your immunity and protect your cells from oxidative damage.

A good source of non-starchy vegetables containing vitamin C are peppers, sprouts, and broccoli. You can easily add peppers to your salad or main dish. Steamed broccoli is also a very healthy option to add to your main dish, serve alongside salmon, or add to your veggie pan salad.

Vitamin E is also helpful in boosting your immune system; it is also essential for your eye health and skin. Carrots, kale, and spinach are options rich in vitamin E that you can easily add to your food. Below are some examples of non-starchy vegetables:

- **Leafy vegetables:** Kale, lettuce, spinach, watercress, cabbage, and Brussel sprouts
- **Root vegetables:** Carrot, turnip, and radishes
- **Squashes:** Cucumber, squash, courgette, and pumpkin
- **Stalk vegetables:** Asparagus, leeks, spring onions, and celery
- **Others:** Broccoli, bean sprouts, mushroom, cauliflower, peppers, and tomato

Vegetables are your best friends. When eaten raw or even when steamed, roasted, or grilled, fresh vegetables can be a very healthy low-carb option. The same applies to frozen vegetables that are lightly cooked. Always opt for low-sodium or unsalted canned vegetables. Canned vegetables with lots of added sodium are not a healthy option.

It is also counterproductive if you eat veggies cooked with lots of butter cheese or a high carb source. If you have hypertension or other diabetes and metabolic syndrome complications, you need to limit your sodium intake, including pickles, etc.

Fatty Fish

Fatty fish are one of the most consistent diet recommendations when it comes to fending off diseases. Some examples are herring, salmon anchovies, mackerel, and sardine.

Salmon contains Omega-3 fatty acids, which have a profound positive effect on your heart health. Taking care of and promoting your heart health helps against the increased risk of heart disease and stroke that people with diabetes are faced with. Studies have shown that several inflammatory markers had dropped when fatty fish was consumed 5 to 7 days per week for about 8 weeks. In addition to all that, it contains high-quality protein and is low in carbs; therefore, it is perfect for maintaining normal blood glucose sugars after meals.

Dairy

Dairy food is a vital food category and with various choices available for you to pick from. Studies have shown that milk product consumption and total dairy products have been associated with a reduced risk of developing type 2 diabetes. It is also protective for those who have prediabetes. The studies were conducted on items from the dairy group, including whole milk and yogurt and total dairy consumption.

Examples of dairy food include milk, yogurt, cream, butter, and cheese. Unsweetened dairy products can be a very healthy choice for those who wish to follow a low-carb diet. There are numerous benefits of dairy foods, as they are a good source of protein, calcium, and vitamin B12. The National Osteoporosis Society recommends that a daily intake of 700 milligrams of calcium is required for adults to maintain healthy bones and other functions that depend on calcium.

Vitamin B12 is an essential source for the nervous system. People with diabetes are at risk of complications of neuropathy that affects the peripheral nerves. Vitamin B12 helps protect against some of the complications of diabetes concerning the nerves. The protein in milk is also essential for muscle repair and growth. The recommended daily intake of calcium can be achieved by just a pint of milk along with another source that includes food such as beans, fish with edible bones like sardines and salmon, and dark green vegetables, for example, kale and broccoli.

For dairy, opt for low-fat dairy; if you want to have high-fat or full-fat dairy, do so but in small proportions. The best choices are skimmed milk, low-fat yogurt, and low-fat or non-fat sour cream or cottage cheese. Some of the worst options are whole milk, regular yogurt, regular sour cream, cottage cheese, and ice cream, etc.

Beans and Pulses

Beans, pulses, lentils, peas, chickpeas, and runner beans are all examples of non-animal sources of protein that can be very beneficial to people with diabetes.

Soya Beans have been included among this group, and it has been supported with research indicating that the consumption of soya beans increases insulin sensitivity and reduces the risk of developing type 2 diabetes.

Adding beans to your salads is a good option for increasing your protein intake.

Fruits to Eat on Low-Carb Diet

Like vegetables, fruits are among the healthiest food groups that you can add to your diet. They are rich in nutrients, especially vitamin C, which helps keep your cells healthy. In addition to the minerals, we also have fiber that aids digestion reducing cholesterol levels. Different fruits have a different combination of vitamins and minerals; for example, grapefruits can be rich in vitamin A and potassium; they can also be rich in vitamin K and manganese.

While fruits have dense nutrients, fiber, and antioxidants, it is important to remember that certain foods have a high glycemic index and can increase your blood sugar levels; therefore, it is essential to be mindful about the types of fruits you eat and when.

Watermelon and Dates

Avoid processed foods, such as apple sauce that have had their fiber removed. If you have a sweet tooth, fruits can be an optimum way to satisfy your desires without compromising your health. Since fruits are high in nutrients and low in fat and sodium, they are optimum if you have obesity or hypertension.

One serving of fruit is a medium-sized fruit that is the size of the piece or a cup of smaller fruits such as berries. You should avoid it, but processed fruits have only half a cup of additives to fulfill the serving size.

Apples

An apple is a versatile fruit that you can snack on raw or cook with some flavoring such as cinnamon or ginger to make a delicious dessert. You can also stuff your apples with some crushed nuts such as walnuts or pecans.

Avocados

Avocados are very high in healthy fats, which are the monounsaturated fats that are beneficial to your body.

Avocados are a tasty option to add to your main dish; slice them along with some salmon or make guacamole.

They're straightforward to prepare or include in any of your dishes.

Berries

Berries are very delicious and versatile fruits. There are strawberries, blueberries, blackberries, etc. There are a lot of things that you can do with berries; for example, you can eat them raw, or you can make them into a smoothie. You can always add various berries to most of your breakfast or snacks, for example, making an oatmeal breakfast or adding mixed berries to your fresh whipped cream or frozen yogurt. They are also rich in antioxidants and very low in calories. They help fight inflammation and other diseases such as cancer.

Citrus Fruits

They are also useful for boosting your immunity; they are loaded with vitamin C. One orange contains all the amount of vitamin C that you require in a day. Since immunity is an issue with people with diabetes, adding citrus foods to your diet is very healthy and a useful low carb option. You can add lemons to your seafood, sauces, or even to your iced water or tea. You can simply make lemons or oranges into a refreshing cold drink. The folate and potassium in oranges help you equalize your blood pressure if you suffer from hypertension. Citrus foods also include grapefruits as well as oranges and lemons.

Peaches

They are juicy and delicious fragrant foods containing lots of nutrients such as vitamins A and C and fiber and minerals such as potassium. They are easy to add to your yogurt or spice them up with some cinnamon or ginger. You can also flavor your tea with peach instead of sugar for a healthy twist on your drinks.

Pears are also tasty treats that you can add up to your salad or snack on. They are rich in fiber and are a good source of vitamin K.

Kiwi is a slightly citrus fruit that is rich in fiber and vitamin C as well as potassium. One large kiwi contains about 13 grams of carbohydrates, which is low carb, making it a delicious yet very healthy option to add to your diet.

Lean Meat

A source of protein that is low in fat and low in calories is lean meat. That means the red meat such as pork chops trimmed with fat or skinless chicken or turkey.

Lean meat is a nutritional protein source for promoting cell health and repair—while also being a low-carb and low-fat option. Poultry is also a rich source of vitamin B3, B6 choline, and selenium. Vitamin B3, which is known as niacin, helps with stress and sex hormones. Erectile dysfunction and stress are an issue for those who have diabetes, and having food with vitamin B3 become very beneficial for people with diabetes. Niacin helps with promoting the nerve functions and can reduce inflammation. Selenium has strong antioxidant properties that help with controlling inflammation and protecting the cells. Selenium also has a role in promoting the immune system, which is very beneficial to people with diabetes.

Red meat is also a rich source of protein, iron, zinc, and vitamin B. Iron is essential for your red blood cells to transport oxygen, as healthy cells require a constant supply of oxygen. Anemia, which is a deficiency in RBCs (Red Blood Cells), can occur due to a lack of iron—which is a condition that could easily be avoided by eating adequate amounts of this mineral. Iron can also be found in dark, green, leafy plants and beans; iron from greens are the best source.

Zinc is also a mineral needed by the body for the synthesis of DNA. It also has a role in helping the immune system to function properly. You can also find zinc in fish eggs and beans, although zinc is better absorbed from fish and meat sources.

Red meat is rich in vitamin B6 and B12. Both help promote the immune system, regeneration, and protection of the nervous system. One medication that some people with diabetes take, known as metformin, causes an increased drop in vitamin B12. Therefore, it becomes necessary to compensate for vitamin B loss from sources such as red meat.

Eggs

Be mindful about the number of eggs you consume, as they can easily raise your cholesterol levels. If you're going to eat an egg, it is preferred to boil and consume the whole egg, as the benefits of eggs line in the nutrients inside rather than the whites. It is a debate whether eggs are helpful or not to people with diabetes due to their low carb content; however, consuming an excessive amount of eggs is associated with increased cholesterol levels. Moreover, apart from being rich in cholesterol, eggs are dense in nutrients, as they have essential fatty acids, proteins, and vitamin D.

Nuts

Nuts that reduce bad cholesterol are very effective because they protect people with diabetes from complications of the narrowing of arteries.

Consuming cashews is very beneficial to lower your blood pressure and decrease the risk of heart disease. They are also low in calories; therefore, they have no negative effect on your blood glucose level. They are also low in fat, so they do not affect your weight negatively. You can have about a handful of cashews every day for the maximum benefit.

Peanuts are rich in fiber and protein, and therefore, they are a beneficial option for people who have diabetes. You can have up to 25 to 30 peanuts every day. You can also roast them. They can control your blood glucose levels.

They are loaded with energy; however, they are good sources of protein and a good source of healthy fats, making you feel full for a long time; therefore, curbing the urge to snack. A study performed showed that eating pistachios was very beneficial to people who have diabetes. Avoid salted pistachios.

Walnuts are high in calories; however, they do not affect your body weight. They have numerous nutritional benefits. Consuming walnuts daily can help in weight loss due to their low-carb content and their possession of substances that activate the fat-burning pathways. They also provoke fasting glucose, which helps you avoid obesity as a complication of diabetes. The high-calorie content helps your body by providing it with energy to don't feel like eating a lot and gaining weight.

Almonds control the blood glucose level and are very beneficial to people with diabetes because they reduce the
oxidative stress that affects cells in diabetics. They are also rich in magnesium. You should avoid salted almonds, but you can also soak them in water overnight to eat them fresh the next day.

How to Tackle Low-Carb Eating?

We don't eat just to relieve physical hunger. For warmth, stress reduction, or to reward oneself, many of us often turn to food. And we prefer to reach out for fast food, candy, and other soothing yet harmful things when we do. When you feel sad, you may reach for a cup of ice cream, order a pizza if you are bored and lonely, or stop by the drive-through after a long day at work.

Emotional eating involves food to help oneself feel better, rather than the stomach, to meet emotional needs. Comfort eating, sadly, doesn't cure emotional issues. Probably, it generally makes you feel worse. Afterward, the initial mental struggle not only persists, but you feel bad about binge eating as well.

It isn't always a negative thing to sometimes use eating as a pick-me-up, a treat, or rejoice. But when food is the main emotional coping method, you get trapped in an addictive loop where the actual feeling or concern is never tackled. Your first instinct is to open the fridge anytime you are depressed, frustrated, furious, sad, tired, or bored.

How you consume is just as or even more significant than what you consume. In emotional overeating, the overall amount of food you consume, your disposition toward eating, how you manage your snacks and meals, and your personal food choices may play a far greater role than the actual foods you want to consume. Take time to evaluate your eating habits, understand more about regular eating vs. emotional eating, and build different self-help methods to resolve both your mental and physical food relationships. Start practicing saying "no," not just to harmful foods but also to circumstances that undermine your attempts to build healthier dietary patterns that are emotionally mindful.

When you're emotionally at the weakest place, the worst food cravings strike. When experiencing a tough situation, feeling depressed, or even feeling bored, you may look to food for warmth—consciously or subconsciously. Comfort eating will undermine your attempts to lose weight. It also contributes to excessive consumption, particularly too much of high-calorie, fatty and sugary desserts. The positive news is that you may take action to retake control of your dietary behaviors and get back on board with your weight reduction plans if you're susceptible to emotional eating.

Recognize Addictive Behavior

Study studies have been dedicated to the issue of food addiction for years, whether or not anyone may be addicted to certain foods, specifically those created with processed goods such as white flour, sugar, salt, and fat, and whether, in turn, these foods were accountable for such habits of bingeing and excessive consumption. As it could not be proved that food itself became addictive, scientists started to look at the habits' addictive features. Addiction components include addictive behavior involvement (such as overeating), lack of control, behavioral preoccupation (eating), having only brief gratification, and permanent detrimental effects (becoming unhealthy or obese from overeating).

Separate Emotional Signals from Hunger Signals

The distinction between feeding in reaction to appetite and feeding in reaction to emotion may be challenging to perceive and recognize. Through feeding mindfully and paying attention to hunger cues, learn to distinguish the two types of feeding and self-regulate your food intake. Practice evaluating your hunger: Exactly how hungry are you on a scale of 1 to 10? If you don't feel hungry or you're only a little hungry, anywhere between one and four, you should rank it. Wait until you hit five, very hungry (but don't let yourself get too hungry to the extent you overeat).

Develop a Schedule

Eating regularly scheduled meals and scheduled snacks for certain persons will deter overeating if you keep to the routine. On the other side, since they lead to random feeding and bingeing, erratic eating patterns typically mean disaster. Generally speaking, at various hours of the day, most people plan three courses and one or two snacks or "micro meals." Typically, true hunger comes in about three hours after the last meal. A tiny snack might be enough at that moment, depending on your eating patterns and the time of day; if not, you get a signal that it's time for your next meal.

Change the Eating Patterns

Some research has shown that missing food, consuming late at night, and other irregular eating habits may contribute to weight gain for some individuals. It doesn't imply that as soon as you wake up the next morning, you can or should have breakfast, nor does it imply that you shouldn't consume something at night. However, it might be time to follow a different pattern if eating habits don't help you shed weight or manage over-eating. Short-term research has also shown that consuming the main meal at noon (for lunch) will promote weight reduction and weight management, rather than later in the day or what might be deemed usual dinner time.

Find Different Ways to Satisfy Your Emotions

You would not be able to regulate your food habits for too long if you don't know how to handle your feelings in a manner that doesn't rely on food. Diets too frequently fail because they provide rational dietary guidance that only works if the food patterns are deliberately managed when feelings derail the system, expecting an instant payoff with food, so it doesn't work.

In order to prevent emotional feeding, you must find other avenues to satisfy yourself psychologically. It's not enough to grasp the emotional eating cycle or even to recognize their causes, even though it's a big first step. For emotional satisfaction, you need substitutes for food that you can resort to.

Several other alternatives to comfort eating are given here:

- Call somebody who always helps you feel good, whether you're sad or lonely, interact with your cat or dog, or glance at a childhood picture or special photo album.
- Release your inner tension if you're restless by listening to your favorite tune, holding a tension ball, or enjoying a fast stroll.
- Give yourself a hot cup of tea if you're tired, take a nap, light some scented candles, or get yourself in a heated blanket.
- Read a good novel, watch a television show, wander in nature, or switch to a hobby that you love (woodworking, guitar playing, playing basketball, jigsaw puzzles, etc.) if you're bored.

Get Social Support

If needed, a community of friends and family, including clinical support in the form of a psychologist or mentor, may be as vital to your progress as your own encouragement and actions. Many that care for your well-being will

 assist by supporting you, exchanging suggestions for healthy foods, acknowledging the social foundations of your unhealthy eating problems, and maybe even helping to solve any of the mental conditions that affect your emotional eating. Surround yourself with friends who are able to lend an ear, give support and inspiration, or maybe join in as buddies for dining, walking, or exercising.

CHAPTER 3:
The Protein Balance

The protein, or amino acids, are used by your body in order to repair damaged tissues, replace old tissues, build muscle, and fight off infections. Thankfully, most people are able to consume protein in the required ranges— neither too much nor too little—without much effort. As long as they eat a few protein-rich ingredients daily, they can achieve the correct amount of protein. The same is not true for people with kidney diseases, who have to be more diligent in managing how much protein they do or don't consume in their diet.

When a person consumes too much protein, it can cause a buildup of excess waste in their blood. As you know, kidney disease results in the kidneys being unable to filter the blood, resulting in excess waste buildup. This means that if a person consumes too much protein when they have kidney disease, they will only be worsening the problem of waste overabundance, and their kidneys will not be capable of handling it. Therefore, it is imperative that people with kidney disease are aware of the amount of protein they consume and that they don't put more than necessary in their meals.

Without amino acids, the body would be incapable of fighting off infections, healing from injuries, and halting excessive bleeding. We would be unable to have any muscle, as well, which would be deadly as the human heart is a muscle itself. This is why it is important to maintain adequate protein intake in your diet. For an average person, protein between forty and sixty-five grams daily is ideal.

There are two types of protein you will consume in your daily diet, which are animal-based proteins and plant-based proteins. A person can choose to consume either a combination of both animal and plant proteins or solely plant-based proteins if they are vegan.

Animal-based proteins are simple to add to your diet, as they contain all of the amino acid building blocks your body requires. This means all you have to worry about is consuming the correct amount of protein. The amount and types of fat found within animal-based protein varies based on the source of the ingredients. For example, steak contains much more fat than chicken breasts. Some animal-based proteins are also higher in saturated fats, which are a less healthy option for heart health. When trying to consume low-saturated fat options for optimal heart health, people typically choose poultry, fish, and reduced-fat dairy options.

Plant-based sources of protein are more versatile in the amino acids they contain. While animal-based proteins contain all the essential amino acids humans require, the variety of amino acids found in most plant-based ingredients is usually reduced. For this reason, if you are relying on plant-based proteins, you will need to ensure you are consuming all nine essential amino acids, which include:

- Lysine
- Isoleucine
- Histidine
- Leucine
- Valine
- Threonine
- Phenylalanine
- Methionine
- Tryptophan

While there are twenty types of amino acids in all, these nine are the most essential to consume in our diets. For this reason, whenever an ingredient contains all nine essential amino acids, it is classified as a complete source of protein. While animal-based products are complete sources of protein, not all plant-based ingredients are. Thankfully, there are still complete sources of plant-based protein, which are important to know about if you are consuming most or all of your protein from plant-based sources. Some examples of complete sources of protein include quinoa, soy, buckwheat, rice paired with beans, and chia seeds. While these are complete sources of protein, you can still get additional amino acids from nuts, grains, lentils, beans, seeds, and vegetables. If people plan their plant-based diet carefully, they can ensure that they are consuming the correct amount of protein needed for their kidney health and the correct amino acids. Plant-based protein sources are also beneficial as they are low in saturated fat, high in fiber, and high in nutrients.

While the exact amount of protein you will need to consume will vary based on the factors we have previously mentioned, frequently, people who are in stages one through three of chronic kidney disease are recommended twelve to fifteen percent of their calorie intake to be protein. If a person is in stage four of chronic kidney disease, this percentage is further reduced, often to being around ten percent of a person's daily caloric intake.

Americans are used to enjoying large servings of protein-rich ingredients, such as meat, fish, and dairy. This can lead to confusion about what you can eat if you have to limit these ingredients to such a degree. This is especially confusing when you consider the fact that you must consume enough calories daily to prevent excessive weight loss and muscle waste. Thankfully, there are healthy ingredients that you can add to your meals to increase their nutrition and bulk up calories. One easy way to do this is by adding olive oil or avocado oil to your meals. These two oils are high in some of the healthiest fatty acids and are high in calories, allowing people to bulk up their calorie content easily.

The exact cause for this improvement with plant-based proteins has not been confirmed. However, there are multiple factors that could be responsible. First, plant-based ingredients are often high in phytonutrients and antioxidants, which have been shown to fight disease and improve overall health. Second, the consumption of these ingredients seems to reduce the production of uremic toxins, which are a type of toxin that is known to worsen the progression of chronic kidney disease and cardiovascular disease.

The third cause of this benefit could lie in the consumption of phosphorus. This mineral, which is known to become overly concentrated in the blood of chronic kidney disease patients, is found in both plant-based and animal-based protein sources. However, the difference is that phosphorus has a different bioavailability rate in both of these sources. While the phosphorus found in animal-based proteins are easily absorbed by the body, the same is not true
 for plant-based protein sources.

Is Optavia Diet Going to Help You Lose Weight?

How much weight you lose following the Optavia diet plans depends on factors such as your starting weight and age, and how well you conform to the plan, and how involved you are.

Optavia reflects the Medifast coach group and lifestyle brand, introduced in 2017. Previous experiments have been carried out using Medifast products and not the current Optavia products. Although the Optavia goods are a new line, Medifast has told the "U.S. News" that they have the same macronutrient profile and are comparable with the Medifast products as well. Therefore, when testing this diet, we assume the following studies are important. There has been no literature conducted directly on the label Optavia.

The studies were limited, with many dropouts, as is true with most diets. Short term, it seems difficult not to lose at least a few pounds; you consume half the calories that other adults consume. Studies appear to back it up. Long term views are less optimistic. Look at the data in more detail here:

A 2017 study funded by Medifast found that by their final visit (anywhere from 4 to 24 weeks later), more than 70% of overweight adults who were placed on Medifast and received one-on-one therapeutic support lost more than 5% of their body mass.

A 2016 research—partially funded by Medifast and published in the journal Obesity—found that obese adults lost 8.8% of their body weight on Medifast products and Optavia-style coaching after 12 weeks, and 12.1 percent of their body weight if they took phentermine at the same time—a weight loss medication that can minimize food cravings.

A research published by "Johns Hopkins Medicine" in 2015 found no credible evidence that most commercial weight loss services, like Medifast, have resulted in long-term weight loss for individuals. The researchers reviewed articles on randomized clinical trials that lasted for 12 weeks or more. In trials lasting 4 to six months, participants in low-calorie meal plans, such as Medifast, lost more weight than nonparticipants. However, the researchers found only one long-term analysis, which at 12 months showed little value to those plans. The researchers also found that the very low-calorie systems carried higher risks of complications, including gallstones.

A 2015 research released in the "Annals of Internal Medicine" reviewed 45 trials, including Medifast, of generic and patented weight-loss programs. Very low-calorie programs, like Medifast, culminated in a weight loss of 4% greater than therapy for four months. But the study found some of this effect lessened after six months of reporting.

A 2015 research in the "Diet Journal" looked at the charts of 310 Medifast overweight and obese clients who followed the "Achieve Plan" and found which participants—who remained on the plan—lost an average of around 24 pounds by week 12 and 35 pounds by week 24. Participants lost more fat than lean muscle no matter their age or gender.

A small research, sponsored and planned by Medifast and published in "Nutrition Journal" in 2010, has randomly allocated 90 obese adults to either the 5&1 plan or a calorie-restricted diet based on government guidelines. Those in the Medifast category had lost a total of 30 pounds after 16 weeks—compared to the other group 14 pounds. But 24 weeks later, the Medifast dieters had recovered more than 10 pounds after dieters steadily upped their calories, while the others had put back on about 2 pounds. The Medifast group at week 40 had less body fat and more muscle mass than at the beginning but did not significantly outperform the control group. Nearly half of the Medifast group and more than half of the control group had ended up dropping out.

A Medifast-funded study of 119 overweight or obese Type 2 diabetics, published in the "Diabetes Educator" in 2008, randomly assigned dietitians to a Medifast diabetic plan or a diet based on "American Diabetes Association (ADA)" guidelines. After 34 weeks, the Medifast group had lost a total of 10 1/2 pounds but had recovered all but 3 pounds after 86 weeks. At week 34, the diabetics on the ADA-based diet lost a total of 3 pounds; after 86 weeks, they'd gained it all back plus a pound. The dropout rate was almost 80%.

What Do You get from These Optavia Diet Recipes?

If you find yourself going off and on a rollercoaster eating habit, you should definitely try out the recipes outlined in this book. Optavia diet comes with the structure and organization needed to get you off on a good start and take you to your desired destination if well-adhered to. Anyway, my friends' account simply portrays that some discipline is, of course, required. Even if you're an emotional eater or a binge eater, the Optavia diet encourages you to exercise a bit of control.

The diet is a high-protein diet that typically makes up about 10–35% of your daily calorie intake. The protein serves as a carb alternative when your body needs energy. On average, your calorie intake per day may hover around 800– 1,000 as the Optavia diet relies on the intense restriction of calories and active promotion of weight loss. The Calories of most of the Fuelings is around 100–110 each.

Optavia diets encourage you to do away with junk by eating nutrition-rich Fuelings and making your own food based on a healthy template. If you are often too busy to cook, the diet allows for a varying degree of flexibility when it comes to preparing your own meal, as well as a complementary degree of pre-packaged foods or Fuelings to go with your cooking timetable. In essence, following the program is a no brainer as a structure that has been provided for you. For individuals seeking to achieve weight loss through healthy eating, the recipes included serve just that purpose, but your eating plan will depend on whether you're watching your weight or trying to reduce your weight. Whatever the case, the plans are simple and detailed. The coaching and community support help you adhere to the structure of the program.

In case you didn't know, the "Fuelings" are the features that make Optavia recipes stand out among many other weight loss programs. The Fuelings are made without artificial additives, colors, or sweeteners. In addition to that, their "select" line is preservative-free. Although the meals are mostly pre-packaged, especially for the first two levels, they still do not contain any stimulants and no wacky pills or supplements. The emphasis is instead placed on regular eating of small portions of meals and snacks each day.

Previous studies by the team at Medifast showed that the Optavia diet might help improve blood pressure in obese people. This is due to the reduction in weight and reduced sodium intake. Research shows that high sodium levels aggravate the risk of high blood pressure in persons with underlying health conditions, especially salt-sensitive individuals. Optavia meal plans generally provide less than 2,300 milligrams of sodium throughout the day. However, this may vary when it comes to the Lean and Green meals, in which case you're at liberty to choose between low and high sodium options. Also, the recipes are simple and easy to make, so you don't have to worry about spending too much time in the kitchen.

What to Buy

Eggs: Eggs are the best source of protein. All kinds of eggs are okay to eat. Normally, egg whites should be preferred, but yolks are fine too.

Chicken Breasts or Cutlets (Skinless): Chicken, like eggs, is a rich source of protein. Buy a good-quality, inexpensive, and lean chicken. You can cook this in a variety of ways. Given that chicken is perishable, always buy it fresh and use it immediately.

Ground Turkey (Lean): Although ground turkey is a bit more expensive, it is a good change when you get bored with eating chicken; you can rely on turkey as a rich source of protein. Once again, you should always buy a fresh turkey and use it immediately.

Steak: Avoid steak if you are on a very strict diet. If not, then you should not miss steak, as it is a good source of protein and fat. Only buy fresh and lean steak.

Mignon Filet: This is very expensive but tasty as well. Buy it occasionally to treat your palate.

Buffalo: This is definitely the most expensive meat on this list. Only buy fresh and lean buffalo meat.

Flounder: Flounder is an inexpensive fish bread that also happens to be very tasty. Buy it fresh as opposed to the frozen variety, but when you have no option, you can go for the frozen ones.

Cod: This is another inexpensive breed of fish that is packed with proteins and is tasty as well.

Pollock: This is a type of lean fish. It is found easily in the seafood section of the supermarket.

Salmon: Salmon is famous for its protein richness and taste. It is also rather fatty, so eat it in moderation. Wild salmon is more expensive than bred salmon.

Tuna (canned): Canned tuna is once again a tasty, inexpensive, and lean fish. However, if you are on a low-sodium diet, you should avoid this fish or eat it in moderation. In addition, only buy fish that is canned in water and not in oil.

Turkey Bacon: Bacon is generally not allowed on a bodybuilding diet, so as a replacement, you should consider buying turkey bacon. Eat it sparingly—twice a month is more than enough as a treat for your taste buds.

Ground Beef (Lean): Buy good-quality, 90% lean beef. It is a high source of protein and can be consumed in the off-season.

Paneer: Paneer is a form of cottage cheese that is popular in the Indian subcontinent. It is slow-digesting, so you can feel full and satiated for a long time. It is versatile, and you can make a variety of things with it.

Pork Tenderloin: Buy good-quality, low-cost, lean tenderloins, as they are a great source of proteins.

Bass (Sea): This is expensive but tasty. You can eat it occasionally.
Swordfish: This is expensive but tasty. You can eat it occasionally.

What Not to Buy

Skinned Chicken: Only buy skinless chicken, as the chicken skin is full of unhealthy fats that are best avoided.

Breaded Chicken: The breadcrumbs add unnecessary carbs to your diet.

Deli Meat: This is full of additives and preservatives and is generally of low quality.

Bacon: As said earlier, avoid bacon. It is tasty but very fatty and, thus, can wreak havoc on your diet plan. This is not good for heart-related issues.

Ground Beef (Fatty): Lean ground beef should be preferred over fatty beef because, as the name suggests, regular beef contains high amounts of fats.

Fatty Cuts of Meat: Go for lean cuts of meats always. Regular cuts generally contain unnecessary fats that are not good for your diet.

Why Optavia Diet Rather Than Other Diet?

Calorie Restriction Impact

Despite the fact that Optavia's eating routine arrangement stresses eating every now and again for the duration of the day—every one of its "Fuelings" just gives 110 calories. "Lean and Green" foods are additionally low in calories.

At the point when you're eating fewer calories, all in all, you may discover the arrangement leaves you ravenous and unsatisfied. You may feel all the more effectively exhausted and even crabby.

Weariness and Isolation at Mealtimes

Optavia's dependence on meal substitutions can meddle with the social parts of getting ready and eating food.

Clients may think that it's clumsy or baffling to have a shake or bar at a family supper time or when feasting out with companions.

How It Compares with others

The Optavia diet can be more viable for fast weight reduction than different plans, basically in view of what a limited number of calories its Fuelings and Lean and Green meals give.

"U.S. News" and "World Report" positioned Optavia as the number 2 best eating routine for quick weight reduction (attached with "Atkins," "keto," and "Weight Watchers").

The 2019 "U.S. News" and "World Report Best Diets" positioned the Optavia Diet 31st in "Best Diets Overall" and gave it a general score of 2.7/5.

Optavia requires less "mental tumbling" than contenders like "Weight Watchers" (for which you need to gain proficiency with an arrangement of focuses) or "keto" (for which you should intently follow and evaluate macronutrients).

Optavia's instructing segment is similar to "Weight Watchers" and "Jenny Craig," the two of which urge members to select in for meetups to get social help.

The exceptionally handled nature of most nourishments you'll eat on the Optavia diet can be a drawback contrasted with the variety of new, entire nourishments you can eat on increasingly independently directed plans, for example, Atkins.

Calorie restriction is essential to weight reduction, and the 5&1 option is particularly conducive to shedding weight rapidly with an 800–1,000-calorie nutritional plan. Carbs also are stored low with a decent amount of protein per serving, which is right for effective weight reduction in maximum instances.

Plus, carb and calorie restriction have shown to have many health advantages, which include advanced glucose metabolism, adjustments in frame composition, reduced danger of cardiovascular chance elements, and other disorder chance elements as nicely.

But the 5&1 plan may not be for anyone, as dropping weight quickly and excessive calorie restriction can be
damaging to your health, and also you virtually won't feel excellent at the same time as muscle loss is likewise an opportunity. 800–1,000 calories are a quite low standard. However, for weight loss, eating 800–1,000 calories can be safe and effective if no longer applied for extended periods.

Research suggests that too few calories can have an effect on metabolism over the years that could make you regain the weight.

But this will additionally be due to long term habits as there are also several different variables to recall in terms of the differences among people. Weight loss isn't continually easy, and retaining it off may be even more difficult; however, it requires everlasting lifestyle changes.

Optavia additionally recommends 30 minutes a day of exercise, which is likewise important for maintaining the weight off and maintaining proper health.

CHAPTER 4:
Optavia Diet in 6 Meals Everyday

Planning before you try to start a diet, the more likely you will be to stick with the diet longer and see immediate results that last. reparationisthe key to nearly all success! The more you can prepare yourself, your kitchen, and your meal

Cleaning out the kitchen is the first step in preparing for a diet. Before shopping for the foods and products, you'll need to start eating Keto, clear your refrigerator, pantry, and cabinets of anything that creates temptation, such as potato chips or ice cream. Other products include:

Processed Foods

- Any food that has sugar or starch listed within the first five ingredients on the nutrition label
- All foods and drinks containing high levels of carbohydrates or sugars
- Sodas, sugary drinks, and juices

Knowing how to shop is one of the most useful skills all diet followers develop as they adapt and become more familiar with how their body reacts to ketosis and what it requires to maintain the state. Here is a look at a sample grocery shopping list put together based on the main ingredients that make up the foundation of a diet and the staples experts and veterans of the diet recommendations for beginners.

Understanding Portion Control

Before we dive into the lengthy details of what the Optavia diet really is and how it works, it is very important first to grasp the whole idea of portion control and the "six-small-frequent-meals" philosophy to lose weight. That is why this first chapter is a comprehensive introduction to the idea of eating smaller meals more frequently throughout the day. We'll start off by introducing the concept of portion control. This would be a great start for people who have never heard of it or never practiced this method of healthy eating and losing weight. Then, we'll get into the significance of it in our daily lives, i.e., why to practice it and what happens if we don't. After that, a section is dedicated to the very many benefits of controlling and limiting our food portions, along with the reasoning and
principles behind the efficacy of six small meals per day. Towards the end, we'll touch upon a very important issue of emotional eating (also known as comfort eating). We'll discuss what it is and what are the different ways to actually practice it efficiently in order to shed pounds and be healthier.

Finally, the very last section will entail some valuable and easy-to-follow tips and tricks to practice portion control for all of you who struggle with the issue.

What Is Portion Control?

Are you having difficulty reducing weight? Even if you make healthy lifestyle decisions like denying candy, exchanging French fries with a Caesar salad, and sweating crazy during the workouts? Do you keep on mounting the scale week in and week out only to see the same persistent figure looking back at you?

The issue may not be what you consume but how much you consume. In reality, portion management is always the most difficult challenge on the road to weight reduction for an individual. If you're looking to reduce, increase, or sustain your weight, maintaining fitness is not only about consuming the right foods but also about having the correct amount of food. This is actually what portion management is: Not eating more (or even less) calories than the body needs. For weight reduction to take effect, one of the very first items discussed in food planning must be portion control.

Portion control is a means of regulating one's consumption by deciding the number of calories in every food serving and restricting intake below a defined level.

The secret to effective weight loss is portion control. Food portion regulation doesn't simply involve having less food, contrary to common opinion, but rather it implies gaining an understanding of how much you consume and the nutrient content of the food. Sticking to one size at a time lets you maintain a balanced nutrient intake from all the various types of foods. Portion control will also help you restrict empty calories while dining out or at a party, making space for healthier options in your day.

In addition to ensuring that you make clean food decisions, portion regulation is often the foundation of a proper diet.

Far too much, without caring about the number of calories we intake, we prefer to eat whatever may be set out on the table in front of us. Loneliness, or intense feelings, such as elation or profound sadness, may contribute to bingeing. It may also result by being confronted with a wide variety of food options. Controlling one's food intake becomes crucial in view of these factors. The emergence of multiple chronic disorders, such as diabetes mellitus, hypertension, excess weight, and unexplained weight loss, may be warded off and managed by sufficient but not unnecessary feeding.

The terms "portion" and "serving" are sometimes used interchangeably by individuals, but servings and portions are not exactly the same amount. And if you are monitoring your calorie consumption and learning food labeling, it counts.

A portion is any quantity of a single food that you chose to place on your plate, while a serving is a prescribed volume of such food based on guidelines on health and diet, such as ChooseMyPlate.gov from the US department of agriculture.

Let's look at an instance here: 1 serving of the cereal and grain category is equivalent to 1 ounce, as per the agriculture department. Not that much. One ounce of white cooked rice is just half a cup or so. The amount of rice you place on your plate might be a lot greater because you may assume you're just consuming one serving of rice while you really consume two or three servings. That's because a half-cup of rice gives your meal about 100 calories, so you may believe you're just consuming 100 calories, but you're really consuming 200 or 300. You will see how the kilocalories will rapidly add up.

Mixing up portions and servings may create confusion, especially when you consume energy-dense foods and high-calorie treats, which can contribute to eating extra calories.

The reference of food portion sizes to ordinary items is a simple way to exercise portion management. For starters, according to the National Institution of Health, a serving of jacket potato is the width of a fist, and one serving of peanut butter is the width of a ping-pong ball.

The more calories you're served, the more you're going to consume, as per the Centers for Disease Control and Prevention. So, turn to smaller dishware as you adapt to consuming smaller servings, which again will render your meals look bigger (and anyway, you feed first with your eyes, right?). This is a minor adjustment that will render the
task a little less overwhelming.

Simply equate the serving amounts of items to common objects—instead of having to remember charts of teaspoons, cups, and ounces. A single serving of different foods as compared to regular objects are the following:

- Fruits and vegetables are around the size of your palm.
- Pasta is around the size of a single ice cream scoop.
- Beef, fish, or poultry should be the size of a card deck or the size of your palms (excluding the fingers).
  Snacks such as nachos or pretzels are around the equivalent of
- cupped nachos.
- A peach is equivalent to the size of a baseball.
- A potato is the equivalent of a mouse of a computer.
- A bagel is compared to the size of a hockey puck.
- A doughnut is compared to the width of a CD.
- Boiled rice should be the width of the wrapping of a cupcake.

Cheese is the size of your entire thumb (from top to bottom) or
- the size of a couple of dices.

Shopping List for Optavia Diet

Breakfast

- 7 oz. spelt flour
- 1 cup coconut milk
- 1/2 cup alkaline water
- 2 tbsp. grapeseed oil
- 1/2 cup agave
- 1/2 cup blueberries
- 1/4 tsp. sea moss
- 1 cup raspberry
- 1/2 tsp. restrained oil
- 1/2 cup sun-dried tomatoes
- 2 cups spinach
- 1/2 cup coarse cornmeal
- 1/2 tbsp. red pepper
- 1/4 cup baking soda
- 1 1/2 cup all purposes flour, divided
- Kosher salt and freshly ground black pepper
- 1 1/2 oz. can drink beer in style
- 1 code and skin without skin
- 1 cup peeled and spread shrimp, large
- 16 percentiles, shake
- 1 lemon, sliced with cedar wedge
  Tartar sauce, mignon, chimichurri, hot sauce, and malt
- vinegar, for cedar
- 1 tbsp. ¾ pant
- 1 tbsp. mustard

Mains

- 1 lb. rib eye steak
- 1 tsp. salt
- 1 tsp. cayenne pepper
- ½ tsp. chili flakes
- 3 tbsp. cream
- 1 tsp. olive oil
- 1 tsp. lemongrass
- 1 tbsp. butter
  1 tsp. garlic powder

Seafood

- ¼ cup chopped fresh cilantro
- ½ cup seeded and finely chopped plum tomato
- 1/3 cup finely chopped red onion
- 10 tbsp. fresh lime juice, divided
- 4–6 oz. boneless, skinless cod fillets
- 5 tbsp. dried unsweetened shredded coconut
- 8 pcs. 6-inch tortillas
- 14 oz. jumbo cooked shrimp, peeled and deveined; chopped
- 4 ½ oz. avocado, diced
- 1 ½ cup tomato, diced
- ¼ cup chopped green onion
- ¼ cup jalapeño with the seeds removed, diced fine
- 1 tsp. olive oil
- 2 tbsp. lime juice
- 1/8 tsp. salt
- 1 tbsp. chopped cilantro

Snacks

- 15 oz. canned white beans, drained and rinsed
- 6 oz. canned artichoke hearts, drained and quartered
- 4 garlic cloves, minced
- 1 tbsp. basil, chopped
- 2 tbsp. olive oil
- Juice of ½ lemon
- Zest of ½ lemon, grated
- Salt and black pepper

Smoothies

- 1 tsp. chia seeds
- ½ cup unsweetened coconut milk
- 1 avocado
- 3/4 frozen burro bananas
- 1 1/2 cups homemade coconut milk
- 1/4 cup walnuts
- 1 tsp. sea moss gel
- 1 tsp. ground ginger
- 1 tsp. soursop leaf powder
- 1 handful kale
- 2 tablespoons extra-virgin olive oil
- 1 onion
- 4 cups fresh baby spinach

- 1 garlic clove, minced
- Zest of 1 orange
- Juice of 1 orange
- 1 cup unsalted vegetable broth
- 2 cups cooked brown rice

Soup and Salad

For the walnuts:

- 2 tbsp. butter
- ¼ cup sugar or honey
- 1 cup walnut pieces
- ½ tsp. kosher salt
- 3 tbsp. extra-virgin olive oil
- ¼ tsp. kosher salt
- 1 head red leaf lettuce, shredded into pieces
- 3 heads endive
- 2 apples
- 1 (8-ounce) camembert wheel

Meat

- 1 lb. beef chuck roast
- 1 fresh lime juice
- 1 garlic clove
- 1 tsp. chili powder
- 2 cups lemon-lime soda
- 1/2 tsp. ssalt
- 2 cups mayonnaise
- 6 plum tomatoes, seeded and finely chopped
- 1/4 cup ketchup
- 1/4 cup lemon juice
- 2 cups seedless red and/or green grapes, halved
- 1 tbsp. Worcestershire sauce
- 2 lb. peeled and deveined cooked large shrimp
- 2 celery ribs, finely chopped
- 3 tbsp. minced fresh tarragon or 3 teaspoon dried tarragon
- salt and 1/4 teaspoon pepper
- 2 cups shredded romaine
- 1/2 cup papaya or peeled chopped mango
- parsley or minced chives

Starches and Grains

- 2 tbsp. extra-virgin olive oil
- 1 onion
- 4 cups fresh baby spinach
- 1 garlic clove, minced
- Zest of 1 orange
- Juice of 1 orange
- 1 cup unsalted vegetable broth
- 2 cups cooked brown rice
- Soup and Salad
- For the walnuts
- 2 tbsp. butter
- ¼ cup sugar or honey
- 1 cup walnut pieces
- ½ tsp. kosher salt
- 3 tbsp. extra-virgin olive oil
- 1 ½ tbsp. champagne vinegar
- 1 ½ tbsp. Dijon mustard
- ¼ tsp. kosher salt
- 1 head red leaf lettuce, shredded into pieces
- 3 heads endive
- 2 apples
- 1 (8-ounce) Camembert wheel

Meal Planner

Meal planning becomes simple in the 5&1 plan when you know the nutritional parameters of a Lean and Green meal according to your lean protein options; a Lean & Green meal contains 5 to 7 ounces of prepared lean protein with three portions of vegetables that are not starchy and up to two portions of healthy fats.

Savor your Lean & Green meal —Whenever it fits best on your timetable, at any time of day If you're eating out or monitoring your consumption, use the "Lean and Green Meal Nutritional Criteria" given below to direct your choices better:

Nutritional Criteria of L&G

Meal Calories: 250–400 Calories, Meal Carbs ≤ 20 grams of total carbohydrates (ideally < 15 grams), Meal Protein >= 25 grams, Meal Fats 10–20 grams. The three key components of each lean and green meal are Protein, good fats, and carbohydrates. The list of ingredients you would need to make a balanced meal and shop according to your meal schedule is provided below.

Protein is classified into the lean, leaner, and leanest types. Purchase groceries according to recipes of your liking and recipe them to your taste.

Leanest: Pick a 7-oz. (the cooked part, which has 0–4 grams of total fat), then includes 2 healthy fat servings. The leanest options are:

- **Fish:** Cod, haddock, flounder, rough orange, tilapia, grouper, haddock, Mahi Mahi, wild catfish, and tuna (canned in water)
- **Shellfish:** Scallops, crab, lobster, shrimp Game meat: buffalo, deer, elk turkey (ground) or other meat around 98% lean
  Meatless choices: 14 egg whites, 2 cups of liquid egg white
- or liquid egg replacement, 5 oz. of seitan, 1 ½ cups or 2 oz. of 1% cottage cheese, 12 oz. of Non-fat (0%) regular Greek yogurt (approximately 15 g carb per 12 ounces)

Leaner: Pick a 6 oz. (the part cooked), which has 5–9 grams of total fat and includes 1 portion of Healthy Fat.

- **Fish species:** Swordfish, halibut, trout, white meat or Chicken breast skin-free turkey (Ground) or other poultry: 95–97% lean meat

- **Turkey:** Light poultry

Meatless choices: Two entire eggs or replacer, 1 ½ cups or 12 oz. of 2% (approximately 15 g carb per 12 oz.)

four egg whites, two entire eggs and one cup of liquid egg cottage cheese, 12 oz. of low-fat (2%) regular Greek yogurt

Lean: Pick a part of 5 oz. Cooked with 10g–20 grams of total fat—no extra portion of healthy fat.

Fish: Tuna (bluefin steak), salmon, catfish farmed, herring, mackerel Lean beef: roasted, ground, steak, lamb pork

fillet or porkchop turkey (ground) or other poultry: 85–94% leaner meat.

Turkey or Chicken (Dark Meat)

Meatless choices: 15 oz. extra-firm or firm (bean curd) tofu, 3 whole eggs who (up to 2 days a week), 4 oz. part-skim cheese or reduced-fat (3–6g fat per ounce, 1 cup shredded), and 8 oz. (1 cup) ricotta part-skim cheese (2–3 g of fat per ounce.) 5 oz. tempe.

Healthy Amounts of Fat

There can be around 5 grams of fats and less than 5 grams of carb in a portion of healthy fat. Include 0–2 Healthy Fat Portions daily depending on your options; for Lean: 1 tsp of oil (any sort), 1 tbsp. of normal, low-carb dressing, for the salad 2 tbsp. lowered-fat, low-carb dressing, 5–10 green or black olives 1 ½ ounce. Avocado ⅓ ounce. Simple nuts, such as almonds, pistachios, or peanuts 1 tbsp. of simple seeds, such as sesame, flax, chia, or Seeds of pumpkin ½ tbsp. regular margarine, butter, or mayonnaise.

Green and Lean Meal: The "Greens" make up a substantial proportion of the carbohydrates eaten in the 5&1 diet. Pick three servings from our Green Choices collection for each of Your meals (Lean& Green). We've sorted the choices for vegetables into the amounts of a lower, medium, and higher carb levels. Every one of them is Acceptable on the Optimum Weight 5&1 meal plan; the list assists You to make responsible choices on food. From the Green

Choice List, pick 3 servings: 1 serving = ½ cup (except where specified) of vegetables with Around 25 calories and around 5 g of carbohydrates. The Greens include low, moderate, and high carbohydrates.

> **Los carb:** 1 cup endive, green leaf lettuce, Butterhead, romaine, iceberg, collard (fresh/raw), spinach (fresh/raw),
> - mustard greens, watercress, bok choy (raw), spring mix ½ cup: cucumbers, radishes, white mushrooms, sprouts (Mung bean, alfalfa), turnip greens, celery, arugula, escarole, Swiss chard (raw), jalapeño (raw), bok choy (cooked), and nopales.
>
> **Moderate Carb:** ½ cup: cabbage, eggplant, cauliflower,
> - fennel bulb, asparagus, Mushrooms, Kale, portabella, summer squash (scallop or zucchini) cooked spinach.
>
> **Higher Carb:** ½ cup: red cabbage, squash, collard, chayote squash(cooked) mustard greens, green or wax beans, broccoli,
> - kabocha squash, (cooked) leeks, Kohlrabi, okra, (any color) peppers, scallions (raw), (crookneck or straightneck) summer squash, Turnips, Tomatoes, Spaghetti Squash, Palm Cores, Jicama, and Swiss (cooked) chard.

Sample Meal Plan Sample

The meal plan of the optimal 5&1 program is very easy and simple to follow. The Fuelings are readily available in pre-packaged and ready to eat from; the only prep you need is for a Lean and Green meal, which is also made easy for you by providing you with the easy recipes and grocery list; a sample meal plan is provided to help you understand the simplicity of this weight loss program. The following are samples of a day on the Optimal 5&1 plan:

- **Sample 1:** Caramel Mocha Shake Fueling
- **Sample 2:** Creamy Double Crisp Peanut Butter Bar Fueling
- **Sample 3:** Roasted Creamy Garlic Smashed Potatoes Fueling
- **Sample 4:** Cinnamon Sugary Sticks Fueling

Sample 5: Chewy Dewy Chocolate Chip Biscuit, Lean and Green meal (your favorite recipe from this book), water intake (check off how many glasses of water you have each day, which should be 8 oz.)

CHAPTER 5:
Weight Maintenance

M a day on this diet. As a result of this approach, the "US News" and "World Report" ranked it second on their lists of the best diets for fast weight loss, but 32nd on its list of the best diets for healthy eating.

Londonost"supplies"containbetween100and110calorieseach,whichmeansy oucanconsumearound1000calories

recognizes that there are other ways to lasting weight loss: "Eat meals and snacks that incorporate lots of products, seeds, nuts, greens, 100% whole grains, eggs, seafood, poultry, greens, low-fat dairy products. Fat, lean meat plus a little indulgence is the best way to lose weight sustainably in the long run." So will the Optavia diet help you lose weight?

The amount of weight you lose after following the Optavia diet programs depends on factors such as your starting weight as well as your activity and loyalty to following the plan. Optavia, launched in 2017, represents the Medifast lifestyle brand and the coaching community. Previous studies have been done using Medifast products, not the new Optavia products. Although the Optavia products represent a new line, Medifast reported to US News that they have an identical macronutrient profile, making them interchangeable with Medifast products. Consequently, we believe that the following studies are applicable to the evaluation of this diet. Little specific research has been published on the Optavia brand. The studies, like most diets, were small, with numerous dropouts. Research seems to confirm this. On the other hand, the long term expectation is less promising.

A Detailed Look at the Data

According to a 2017 Medifast-sponsored study, more than 70% of overweight adults who received individual behavioral support and underwent Medifast have lost more than 5% of their body weight since their last visit, which is four to 24 weeks.

According to a 2016 study published in the journal Obesity and with partial support from Medifast, obese adults lost 8.8% of their body weight after 12 weeks with Optavia-style training and Medifast products, and also 12,1% of your bodyweight if you were taking phentermine at the same time, which is a weight-loss drug that can reduce binge eating.

However, the researchers found only one long term study, which indicated no benefit for these 12-month plans. The researchers found that there is also an increased risk of complications such as gallstones on ultra-low-calorie programs.

However, the study found that the effect was reduced beyond six months of reporting the results.

During a small study—designed and funded by Medifast and published in 2010 in the Nutrition Journal, —90 obese adults were randomly assigned to either the low-calorie diet or the 5&1 plan according to government guidelines. The Medifast dieters, however, regained more than 4.5 kilograms 24 weeks later, after the calories gradually increased. The others gained only 2 pounds. Compared to the initial exercise, the Medifast group had more muscle mass and less body fat at week 40, but it did not outperform the control group. Eventually, about half of the Medifast group and more than half of the control group withdrew.

According to a Medifast-funded study of 119 overweight or obese type 2 diabetics published in Diabetes Educator in 2008, dieters were randomly assigned to either a Medifast diabetes plan or a diet based on the recommendations of the American Association of Diabetes. After 34 weeks, the Medifast group had lost an average of 4.5 kilos but regained almost 1.5 kilos after 86 weeks. Over 34 weeks, those who followed the ADA-based diet lost an average of 3 pounds; they got everything back plus an extra pound in 86 weeks. By the end of the year, about 80% had given up.

According to an analysis funded by Medifast and published in 2008 in the journal Eating and Weight Disorders, researchers analyzed the medical records of 324 people who were on a diet, were overweight or obese, and were also taking a prescribed appetite suppressant. In 12 weeks, they lost an average of 21 pounds; in 24 weeks, they weighed 26 1/2 pounds and 27 pounds in 52 weeks.
 Furthermore, for approximately 80% of them, at least 5% of the initial weight had been lost in all three evaluations.

This is great if you are obese because losing just 5–10% of your current weight can help prevent some diseases.

However, these numbers are accompanied by some asterisks. First, because they are based on people who completed the 52-week program, they were more likely to lose weight (weight loss was still effective but less pronounced in a cessation analysis).

Second, a review of patient data is given less importance than a study with a control group. Finally, in a survey in which researchers divided dieters into consumer groups on Medifast, that is, those who recognized that they consume at least two shakes a day at each check-in and those who are inconsistent, it is said the rest; the weight losses of the two groups were not significantly different. The Optavia diet has generated headlines throughout the year. Users must enroll in a low-calorie meal plan and then purchase the pre-packaged foods that are part of the chosen plan. In this sitemap, no food group is completely off-limits promising "permanent transformation, one healthy habit at a time."

Although it has many fans, Optavia is not cheap. The US News and World Report ranked it second in the rapid weight loss category. In 2018, it was also a popular diet on "Google." The famous "cake chef" Buddy Valastro credits Optavia for his recent weight loss.

Do you want to try the Optavia diet? Will this really help you lose weight? Here's everything for you: the health implications if they are difficult to follow and the likelihood of reaching your weight loss goal.

How to Maintain Weight

Keeping weight down requires losing weight slowly and steadily, and most of all, being consistent with the Eating Right schedule and workout program. After making some simple changes in eating choices and adding consistent exercise, most of you will lose approximately 3–4 pounds the first week. Then, a weight loss of approximately 1 pound per week can be expected. It is important to do some sort of exercise each day, whether it is weight training, taking a Yoga, Pilates, or Aerobics class, or simply walking. Exercise is critical. Think about this formula:

Eating Right + Exercise

Successful dieters do CHEAT—so plan a cheat day! It means you can choose a day to eat whatever you want at every meal or all day and simply return to your regular healthy eating habits the very next day. Be warned! Cheating on a decadent meal, for example, will make the body rebel. No matter how wonderful the food tastes going down, once the body has adjusted to eating with the proper balance of good healthy food, the shock of those excess calories, fat, and sugar will be difficult to tolerate.

If it is not a cheat day, and the need for something forbidden is felt, treat yourself to a low-fat version or, instead of eating fattening food, purchase a new workout outfit. Looking good and feeling good when you exercise makes it more fun! Learn to treat yourself without using food. Find a special place to alleviate stress. Seek surroundings that are peaceful and beautiful for you. Take time to be pampered.

There is so much pressure on women to look like the women who grace the fashion magazines and are in the endless array of infomercials and television shows. Have you asked yourself—how do they do it? How do they stay slim and fit? It takes more than scheduling workouts at the gym and gulping down a mug of coffee on the way to work. It will not sustain you for very long.

Here are some suggestions for staying slim and healthy at the same time:

Stick to Your Routine: This means, find foods that work for you and will keep you full without increasing your waistline. You have to take the guesswork out of eating your meals, especially breakfast and lunch. It might be scrambled egg whites with vegetables every morning and a grilled chicken salad for lunch—EVERY DAY! You might change the ingredients just a bit by making an omelet instead or substituting salmon for grilled chicken. Develop a routine that makes Eating Right a HABIT rather than a daily BATTLE.

Eat Something Before Going out to a Party: Going out to dinner or to somewhere that is a part of life, and if you eat well during the day, it will allow you a little room when ordering off the menu.

Know What to Do at Parties: All those delicious dishes at parties can pack on the pounds faster than you may think, so make a point of holding a clutch purse in one hand and a glass of wine in another hand—that way, you do not have any hands free to nibble.

Always Take Food with You When You Travel: Do not go anywhere without food. You can always find a piece of fruit, nuts, or a protein bar, so when the cart starts coming down the aisle with nothing but processed foods, it makes it easier just to order water with lemon or tomato juice.

Do Not Allow Yourself to Get Hungry: Before you start feeling those pangs of hunger, take some time to eat ½ of a protein bar, and take your time eating it. It takes a little while for your body to register that it is full and satisfied, so do not rush it!

Exercise: No matter what, find time in your day to exercise. Wake up every morning and figure out when you can exercise by taking a Pilates class or doing Yoga or lifting weights, or getting on the treadmill. MAKE EXERCISE A PRIORITY and NOT AN OPTION. Would you think of going through a day without brushing your teeth or taking a shower? Think about making the time to exercise and find something you enjoy doing and look forward to, even if it is only 20 minutes of Yoga, for example.

Consistency Is the Key: Do whatever it takes to stick with your plan. There are always going to be distractions or issues that arise, so always have a Plan B.

Treat Yourself: If you are going to CHEAT, indulge in foods that are totally worth it. If you really want dessert, the low-fat version doesn't always fit the bill or satisfy the craving. Instead, have a small portion of the 'real' thing. You will find that you appreciate it more when you have it in moderation.

Tips for Weight Maintenance

Here are a few of the tips you can use to practice controlling your portions to lose weight:

Measure Portions to Avoid Overeating

Portion regulation helps with an appreciation of serving quantities through consuming only the proper quantity of every food. As a guide, use the "Nutrition Facts" table used on all pre-prepared items. The serving size, accompanied by the number of servings contained in the package, is the first entry. Much of the details below depend on the quantity of food in a single serving, like carbohydrates, fats, and sodium. If you consume double the serving size, you have double the amount of calories, carbohydrates, and fats mentioned. Measure the snack or count the number of cookies where possible, for instance, and be sure you don't consume further than you planned.

You have to weigh them in order to understand the exact portions of food. Measuring containers and bowls can aid, but overfilling a cup or bowl can be simple. Using a modern food scale, the most effective way to calculate meals is by weight.

Serve Your Food on a Plate

Placing the meals on a plate instead of consuming out of the tub, jar, or served dish is another perfect way to maintain portion sizes. Fill half of your dish with lettuce and vegetables for dinner and lunch, and then split the other half into proteins and carbohydrates. If you have to look for a second portion, you can overeat less frequently.

Limit Nibbling on Food while You're Preparing it

You ought to give up grazing in order to consume fewer. It's enticing to taste the food while you're preparing it, but it's best to wait before the dinner is made. By the same point, it's tempting to neglect to count calories that were not on your own plate, so avoid taking leftovers from the plate of your kid or partner. You will broaden your mind to the excess calories you gain in a day by maintaining a food journal. For a few days, write down any bite you take or drink you sip, and then read the list. The findings may shock you and promote better dietary behaviors.

Don't Bring Extra Food onto The Table

Set aside any food that won't be placed on your plate once you settle down to eat. If you had to pull the food out once again, you would be less motivated for a further serving. Even overeating may be induced by only having food lying inside arms reach. Concealing leftover food, quick snacks, and sweets somewhere you can't see them all the time will help you consume little.

Split the Food

Owing to the large serving sizes that restaurants offer, dining out is a significant contributor to bingeing. Try consuming just half the food the next time you head out. You'll conserve half the amount of calories. By packing up some extra portion of "to go" before you even feed, you may ask your waiter to help. Dividing a meal with a mate is
 yet another simple and inexpensive way to consume less.

Include More Veggies

If you are going to overeat something, the safest way is to eat vegetables. Next, load your bowl with veggies with a minimum of five servings a day. Veggies are easier to afford and very low in fat and calories, but high in fiber as well as other phytonutrients and phytonutrients. That's very effective in helping you preserve good fitness. When it comes to loading the plate, nutritionists advocate concentrating on non-starchy vegetables.

Consume as much Caesar salad as you want to spice up the meal (such as kale, broccoli, tomato, celery, and zucchini). Include herbs for flavor, but retain the prescribed portion size with fats, protein, and carbohydrates. A perfect way to fuel up without eating more calories is to incorporate more veggies into your recipes. Begin your dinner with lettuce, finish your lunch with vegetables and carrots, and add your morning eggs to your preferred steamed veggies.

Use Plates That Are Smaller

Over the decades, when plate dimensions have risen, so have food portions. To hold portions in control, pick 9-inch plates for grownups and 7-inch plates for kids. Your plate will appear fuller; your subconscious will be fooled into believing that you have more fuel.

Always Listen to Your Body

We're all guilty of multitasking. Try to stop feeding when watching TV or while you're on the phone. Studies suggest that mindless consumption contributes to excess weight, so make sure to calculate the right portion sizes and actually consume your treats from a bowl.

It sounds so easy, but in reality, many of us let our minds rule our bodies rather than the other way around, particularly when it comes to emotional eating. Ask yourself whether you're very hungry before getting a snack or whether you're listening to your desires or feeding out of habit. Consume less by not using eating to cope or distract you; instead, take a stroll. And don't just grab a bag of snacks while you're watching a movie or buy popcorn while you're at the cinema.

Be Smart About Salads

Thought food portions for salads wouldn't count? Often remember, it's good to be aware of your chopped vegetables and portions as much as for other meals. For optimum eating and a healthy mix of ingredients, figure out how to make the best of your next salad.

Drink Water Before Eating

Do not forget to consume a ton of water prior to eating before you get to sort your meals. One of the easiest strategies is to drink a glass of water half an hour before a meal or whatever you snack. This is because you're more apt to consume extra while you're dehydrated. It ensures you get more water throughout from getting a huge glass of water, but you're still less likely to get that large of a portion amount.

Use a Plate or Your Palm as a Guide

Use the plate or palm guideline to get a sense of the quantity of starch, calories, fats, and vegetables to have in a serving. Divide the portion into half a dish of low-starch vegetables, a fifth of a plate of protein, a fourth of a plate of complex carbohydrates, and half a tablespoon of fat. Use the palm to 'measure' out reasonable quantities, and use it in combination with the plate principle.

Note to maintain the size of your hand's palm for protein, your finger's tip as a butter serving size, a fourth of an avocado per serving, and no more than the width of a matchbox to measure cheese.

Use the Same Plates and Bowls

Think about it: when it's placed on a large plate, a regular pasta serving seems even smaller, implying that after eating, we're more inclined to feel dissatisfied. Whether the plate is rather big or tiny, or whether the bowls are wider than you've had before, it's very simple to get a bit confused in your mind. You assume you have the same quantity; however, you're having more because of the illusion of the portion.

Change Your Spoon Size

Admit it; you eat more than soup with your oversized spoons. Okay, it's time to quit the trend because evidence suggests that we consume fewer if we use a teaspoon instead of a tablespoon, according to experts. So, if possible, pick a smaller scooper, specifically when it comes to calorie-rich snacks like ice cream.

Another Pro Tip: Consider switching the broad serving spoons too; it's tougher to put on huge quantities with a smaller version.

Eat Slowly and Savor

Eating quickly makes you more apt to skip the hunger and fullness indicators. Taking your time with a meal, actually treasuring each taste, encourages you to experience the meal further and can ensure that you don't overeat what you're consuming. This implies not pacing in front of the TV, over the countertop, or gulping down the dinner. Sit and eat mindfully and frequently. Eating quickly and in a rush, food will feel less enjoyable.

Mind to ensure your foods are balanced in terms of macro and micronutrients, a source of nutrition, good fats, and complex carbs to make these portion-controlled meals more fulfilling. Have low GI (gastrointestinal) effects with carbohydrates, such as lentils, chickpeas, beans, brown rice, quinoa, and butternut squash. They're all excellent energy sources you absorb slowly and offer you energy for a long period. Include healthier fats, such as avocado, almonds, nuts, and olive oil because the fat makes us remain fuller, plus it's very nice for your skin, hair, and body. And, of course, high-quality poultry, such as meat, sustainably captured salmon, and leaner varieties of grass-fed beef and lamb if necessary. This aims to enhance the quality of the fatty acids found in the meat. Add more legumes, tofu, and kimchi for vegetarian forms of protein. Not only is stuff like lentils (chickpeas, lentils) a decent supply of carbs, they add up and are also a very nice source of protein.

Conclusion

The program has earned worldwide acclaim for its ability to deliver sustainable results without complicating the meal program for people. It places very few restrictions on food and inspires people to choose a healthier version of their daily food without compromising taste or nutrition.

Choosing the right diet or program had also become difficult as the industry flourished. Many diets claim to have specific health problems while helping a diet lose weight.

Unlike other diets, the Optavia diet is not designed for a specific health condition. It is designed according to the dieters' needs to achieve the ideal weight and the healthy lifestyle you want.

When you desire a structure and need to lose weight rapidly, the Optavia diet is the perfect solution.

The extremely low-calorie eating plans of the Optavia diet will definitely help you shed more pounds.

Before you start any meal replacement diet plan, carefully consider if it is truly possible for you to continue with a specific diet plan. When you have decided to stick with Optavia and make progress with your weight loss goal, ensure you have a brilliant knowledge about optimal health management to enable, and archive desired results effortlessly in the shortest time period.

The Optavia diet program is a stress-free and easy-to-follow program. It is a cool way to start a journey to your health.

Thank you!

Ketogenic Diet

Text Copyright © Author

Legal & Disclaimer

The information contained in this book is not designed to replace or take the place of any form of medicine or professional medical advice. The information in this book has been provided for educational and entertainment purposes only.

The information contained in this book has been compiled from sources deemed reliable, and it is accurate to the best of the Author's knowledge; however, the Author cannot guarantee its accuracy and validity and cannot be held liable for any errors or omissions. Changes are periodically made to this book. You must consult your doctor or get professional medical advice before using any of the suggested remedies, techniques, or information in this book.

Upon using the information contained in this book, you agree to hold harmless the Author from and against any damages, costs, and expenses, including any legal fees potentially resulting from the application of any of the information provided by this guide. This disclaimer applies to any damages or injury caused by the use and application, whether directly or indirectly, of any advice or information presented, whether for breach of contract, tort, negligence, personal injury, criminal intent, or under any other cause of action.

You agree to accept all risks of using the information presented inside this book. You need to consult a professional medical practitioner in order to ensure you are both able and healthy enough to participate in this program.

Table of Contents

Introduction

Many people would say that they got fat because they got lazy and started to eat more. But what if it was the other way around? What if those people just got fat and simply became less active which led to them eating more?

For the past several decades we have been provided advice about nutrition that has been found to be inaccurate, at best. At worst, some of that information has proven to be entirely false. Nutritionists and physicians *know* that some studies from the 1950s to today have been severely manipulated. The reason being that many of these studies received funding from companies that produce foods and food additives that are not good for us. These studies build the foundation of the food pyramid that has been taught in schools since the 1960s and has led us to what we have been told is a 'balanced diet'.

Originally developed in 1924 by Dr. Russell Wilder at the Mayo Clinic, the ketogenic diet was very effective in the treatment of epilepsy that didn't respond to the current medications for that disease. Despite the studies showing how effective the diet was in treating epilepsy, especially in young children, it fell out of favor after the discovery of new anti-seizure medications in the 1940s.

The ketogenic diet is very closely related to the paleolithic diet which also excludes most carbohydrates. Unfortunately, today's diet consists of a high level of carbohydrates which cause significant changes in our health. Carbohydrates are by far the most fattening ingredient in our diets – even beyond the amount of pure fat we consume.

The ultimate goal of following a low-carbohydrate ketogenic diet is to improve your heath by making your body burn ketones rather than glucose for energy. Within this book you will learn what the ketogenic diet is and how it works, things you should know and do before starting this diet plan, and how to make it work for you.

By following a balanced ketogenic diet, you can feel good in your own skin again! You'll have more energy, your skin and hair will be smoother and more healthy, not to mention the reduction of stress, depression and anxiety that can nag you as you go about your day.

Chapter 1:

What is a Ketogenic Diet?

Quite literally, the ketogenic diet is a high-fat, moderate-protein, low-carbohydrate diet that was originally used to treat epilepsy in children who did not respond well to the medicines available at that time.

This diet forces the body to burn fats for energy rather than carbohydrates. The body converts the carbohydrates in our food into glucose which is then sent throughout the body to be used as energy. Unfortunately, if you take in more carbohydrates than you need for the amount of energy you use during a day the excess glucose is converted to fat and stored rather than being eliminated. However, if you restrict the amount of carbohydrates ingested, the liver will begin converting fat into fatty acids and ketone bodies. Once ketones in the blood outnumber the molecules of glucose, the cells of your body will begin using those ketones as their source of energy.

How Does a Ketogenic Diet Work?

The ketogenic diet shifts the body's metabolism from utilizing glucose as energy to ketones. While it doesn't guarantee instant weight loss, it is an effective tool to help you reach your goals of living healthier.

First, you are going to be eating very satisfying and nutritious foods that will make you experience fewer cravings and be hungry less often. Today's nutritionists won't tell you that *good* fats cause satiation, **not** fruits and veggies. It has been determined through medical studies that protein and fats are the most satisfying of the three macronutrients you will be concerned with when following this new lifestyle.

Second, eating fats actually helps your body burn the fat you already have stored so that you can lose weight a bit more easily. Carbohydrates cause the body to produce insulin to move glucose molecules into the cells to be used for energy. Unfortunately, nearly everyone who is overweight for a long period of time will experience some form of insulin-resistance even if they have not been diagnosed as diabetic. This means that you will experience both high and low blood sugar levels as well as more cravings.

And third, you will be able to achieve greater weight loss due to the metabolic advantage the low-carbohydrate diet supports. When your liver break fats down there are always more ketones than your body can actually use so the excess is excreted through urination. However, that loss of potential energy is not too great so you won't even miss it.

How Does a Ketogenic Diet Compare to 'Traditional' Diets?

You may have tried one or two – or many – of the more traditional diets and had a couple weeks to a few months worth of weight loss but found it very easy to ... let's say, fudge your diet? And I mean that literally – fudge can be a big downfall. Am I right?

Compare the following two lists and see how the ketogenic diet can help you achieve your weight-loss goals.

Traditional Diet

- Restricts fat intake

- Allows for moderate protein intake

- Increases fruit and vegetable intake

- Follows Food Pyramid guidelines

- Restricts caloric intake

- Doesn't allow adjustments to reduce excess hunger

- Doesn't alleviate cravings

- May require purchasing specially packaged meals depending on what diet is being followed

Ketogenic Diet

- Restricts carbohydrate intake

- Allows for moderate protein intake

- Increases beneficial fat intake

- Flips the Food Pyramid guidelines on its head

- Restricting caloric intake is not *absolutely* necessary

- Allows adjustment to reduce excess hunger
- Alleviates most, if not all, cravings

- Doesn't require specially purchased foods unless you choose to do so

As you can see, the ketogenic diet is the total opposite of any traditional diet you may have tried. Maybe that's why it works so well.

Is the Ketogenic Diet Dangerous?

You may have heard that the ketogenic diet is dangerous to your health. Even doctors have been known to say this same thing. However, these 'dangers' are merely myths passed on by people who have a limited understanding of low carb diets and how they work.

One of the main criticisms is that because it's *a high fat diet that it will cause you to have a higher chance of heart related problems.* The message that fat is what makes you fat has been drummed into the collective consciousness of Americans for the last 30 years or more. This message has been repeated over and over again but it is a lie. It's very difficult to unlearn a lie that you've been taught for most, if not all, of your life. The reality is that a high carb diet drives up your blood sugar and insulin levels. Sugar and insulin causes inflammation in your body. The fats allowed on the ketogenic diet are saturated fats and while saturated fats are healthy for you, when combined in the standard American diet it gets the blame for causing heart disease. This is because it was studied in combination with a high carbohydrate diet. The ketogenic diet, which is high in saturated fat and very low in carbohydrates, will actually reduce inflammation because of the reduction of glucose and insulin in your body.

Another criticism is that *high intake of saturated fats and cholesterol causes heart disease.* This is another lie that has been perpetuated for multiple decades. A study from Johns Hopkins Medical School says that the ketogenic diet is healthier **because** of the higher saturated fat intake. Higher saturated fat intake increases HDL (good) cholesterol. At the same time, the lower carbohydrate intake decreases triglyceride levels. These are the two factors that are the markers for heart disease; the closer your triglyceride and HDL levels are to 1, the healthier your heart. It is known that heart disease is caused by consuming a high level of carbohydrates on a daily basis rather than a high saturated fat consumption.

A third criticism is that *people don't do well in ketosis*. This isn't entirely true. As will be discussed later in this book, you should consult with your physician before starting a ketogenic diet plan and if you have certain pre-existing medical conditions then you should either avoid the lifestyle or be strictly supervised my your medical care provider. However, it has been found that our caveman ancestors survived in a state of constant ketosis because grains were very difficult to gather in large quantities and the grains they did gather were not as highly processed as the carbohydrates consumed today.

Yet another criticism, potentially the most damning but least likely to occur, is that *there is the danger of a person following the ketogenic diet to fall into ketoacidosis.* Ketoacidosis is a life-threatening condition but simply being in ketosis is not enough to cause you to develop this condition. Ketoacidosis occurs when there is an abnormally high level of ketones in the blood brought on by an **unregulated** biochemical reaction. This generally occurs in people diagnosed with Type 1 diabetes who cannot produce insulin on their own. Nutritional ketosis is a regulated process that allows enough insulin to remain in the blood to counteract the level of ketones which will prevent a nominally healthy individual from developing ketoacidosis. The only ways for someone following the ketogenic diet to develop ketoacidosis are:

1. If they are in starvation mode for several months. This will not occur with a properly formulated meal plan.

2. If they perform prolonged periods of extremely high intensity exercise.

3. If they are chronic alcoholics who indulge in extreme binges.

As you can see, nutritional ketosis is not dangerous when a properly formulated and followed ketogenic meal plan is in place. It is a natural metabolic process that is perfectly safe for anyone who is not a diabetic who lacks insulin or a severe alcoholic.

Chapter 2:

What Should I Know & Do Before Starting?

A s with any diet, there are a few things that you should know and do before starting.

First and foremost, be patient with yourself. You may experience side effects as you alter your metabolism. You may also experience initial rapid weight-loss followed by a plateau. Just don't be discouraged, it's just your body adjusting to the new amount and type of energy being provided.

Second, talk to your physician to be certain that beginning a specialized lifestyle such as the ketogenic diet is for you. You don't want to endanger your health in the process of trying to improve it.

And third, understand what you may experience and how to ease any symptoms you may have to deal with.

Check With Your Physician

Most medical doctors are not trained in nutrition and probably don't understand the differences between nutritional ketosis and ketoacidosis. While ketoacidosis *is* life-threatening it is very rare that it occurs in people not diagnosed with Type 1 diabetes, who are unable to produce insulin.

There is a great deal of misleading information out there that has been taught since the 1950s and 1960s. Most medical professionals tend to not offer advice that is the opposite of what is generally accepted. If this is the case with your physician, don't be surprised if they can't find a reason (other than your new lifestyle) for your weight loss and overall health improvement.

Who Should Not Follow a Ketogenic Diet?

While the ketogenic diet has been shown to be safe for nearly everyone to follow, there are still certain people who **should not** follow this lifestyle. The first list is rather technical but it will help your physician determine if this lifestyle is healthy and safe for you.

People with Metabolic Conditions

- Type 1 Diabetes

- Primary Carnitine Deficiency

- Carnitine palmitoyltransferase (CPT) Type 1 or 2 deficiency

- Carnitine translocase deficiency

- Beta-oxidation defects

- Mitochondrial 3-hydroxy 3-methylglutaryl CoA synthase (mHMGS) deficiency

- Long-, Medium-, & short-chain acyl dehydrogenase deficiency (LCAD), (MCAD), & (SCAD)

- Long- & Medium-chain 3 hydroxyacyl-CoA deficiency

- Pyruvate caboxylase deficiency

- Porphyria

People with certain Medical Conditions

- Pancreatitis

- Gall Bladder disease

- Impaired liver function

- Malnutrition

- Gastric bypass surgery

- Abdominal tumors

- Impaired gastric motility (this can be due to cancer treatment and medications)

- Kidney failure

- If you are pregnant or breastfeeding

Pros & Cons of the Ketogenic Diet

Changing your eating habits to the ketogenic diet is not easy at first. However, once you are adapted to this new lifestyle you will find yourself feeling much better and healthier as a result. Remember that these side effects are only temporary and will last from a few days up to about a month. If you understand your physical reactions you will be able to find a way to minimize them which will keep you from some of the misery caused by carbohydrate withdrawal.

Let's get the bad news over with before we go on to the benefits of following the ketogenic diet.

Side Effects

- Frequent urination

- As you begin to burn up the stored glycogen in your body, your kidneys will begin getting rid of excess water. For every gram of glycogen stored in your muscles, 3-4 grams of water is also stored. That's a lot of water to get rid of.

- Fatigue, Dizziness, Muscle Cramps & Headache

  - As you begin to excrete excess water it is a given that you will lose electrolytes as well; sodium, potassium and magnesium.
  - Fatigue and dizziness are more common of the side effects but can be avoided by getting enough replacement electrolytes.
  - Using sea salt to season your food along with a lite salt that is potassium based will help you to replace those minerals you are losing.
  - 400mg Magnesium citrate supplements every night before bed will keep you from developing muscle cramps.
- Hypoglycemia

  - Also known as low blood sugar.

  - If you've been eating a high carbohydrate diet your body is used to a certain amount of insulin floating around in your bloodstream. When you reduce your carbohydrate intake you may experience a few episodes of low blood sugar before your body adapts to the new lifestyle.

- Constipation

  ○ Constipation is another of the more common side effects of the ketogenic diet. It is usually due to dehydration and salt loss though it can also be due to eating too many nuts or a magnesium imbalance.

  ○ This can be alleviated by balancing your calcium intake, drinking more water and cutting back on the amount of nuts you consume.

- Sugar Cravings

  ○ There is a 2 day to a 3 week transition period where you may find yourself experiencing intense sugar cravings. How long this side effect will last is dependent upon how long and how much carbohydrate you consumed.

  ○ You can ease these cravings by doing one of the following things:

    ▪ Eat 4 ounces of protein.

    ▪ Take a walk.

    ▪ Take a B Complex vitamin.

- Distract yourself. Sugar cravings last about an hour so if you can take your mind off it, you will be able to outlast the craving.
- Diarrhea

  ◦ This side effect is not unusual and will resolve itself after a few days.

  ◦ Take an anti-diarrheal or use a teaspoon of sugar-free Metamucil just before your meals until the loose stools stop occurring.
- Sleep Changes

  ◦ This side effect varies from person to person.

  ◦ It may be an indication that you are experiencing reduced insulin or serotonin levels. It can also be an indication of a histamine intolerance.
  ◦ If you find yourself not able to stay asleep, you can try eating a snack just before bed containing protein with a little carbohydrate in it.
  ◦ You can also try taking a melatonin supplement to help you fall and stay asleep.

- Kidney Stones

  ◦ Kidney stones are very rare in people following a ketogenic diet. However, it is necessary to mention it just in case you are one of the rare folks who experience this side effect.

- ○ Be sure to speak to your doctor before taking any potassium citrate supplement if you have kidney or blood pressure problems.

- Low T3 Thyroid Hormone levels

    - ○ This isn't actually a bad side effect. It's more a mention of a natural consequence of getting into ketosis. It happens with the more traditional diets as well.
    - ○ Your body will become more sensitive to the T3 hormone levels so you don't need as much.

- Heart palpitations

    - ○ There are several reasons why you might experience this side effect.

        - You may have a normally low blood pressure.

        - You may need a multivitamin with selenium and zinc as well as a magnesium supplement.

        - It may be due to transient hypoglycemia.

        - You may have an electrolyte imbalance or be dehydrated.

- You may be consuming too much MCT oil such as coconut oil. You should include butter, olive oil and animal fats as well.
- You may need a higher protein intake. Try adding an additional 5-10 grams to your diet.

- Hair loss

  - This side effect isn't related just to the ketogenic diet. It is possible with any major change in your diet.
  - Once your insulin levels normalize the hair loss will stop and you should begin to find your hair to be thicker and fuller as it becomes healthier.

Benefits of Going Keto

- Lack of hunger

  - Ketones decrease your appetite.

  - Beneficial fats are very satisfying.

  - You may find yourself forgetting to eat which may be amazing if you struggle with food addiction.
- Lower blood pressure

- Be sure to consult with your doctor if you are taking any blood pressure medications since you may feel dizzy from too much medicine while on the ketogenic diet.
- Lower cholesterol levels

  - Cholesterol is made from excess glucose so when you eat fewer carbohydrates your cholesterol levels will drop.
  - Increased HDL levels also occur because you will be eating more saturated fats, which is a good thing.
  - Decreased triglycerides will occur because they are closely tied to the amount of carbohydrates you consume.
- Lower blood sugar and insulin levels

  - With less sugar coming in, less insulin will be floating in your bloodstream.

  - HbA1c will also decrease which indicates you are at less of a risk for heart disease.

- Increased energy

  - Even if you experience fatigue as a side effect, once you adapt to the ketogenic diet you will find the chronic fatigue symptoms abating.
- Less stiffness and joint pain

- This is one of the best side effects you will experience by following the ketogenic diet.

- It is known that grain-based food increases inflammation and causes many chronic illnesses that overweight people suffer from.

- Reduced 'fogginess'

  - Since the brain is at least 50% fat by weight, it makes sense that the more fat you eat the better your brain can maintain itself.

- Stabilized sleep patterns

  - Sleep apnea has been linked to grain consumption as well as the heartburn that can be caused by a high carbohydrate diet.
  - You will no longer feel the need for those late afternoon naps that can mess up your circadian rhythm.

- Weight loss

  - This is the most common side effects of following a ketogenic diet.

  - As your metabolism repairs itself you will find yourself dropping pounds and inches as you get healthier in the process.

- After the initial rapid weight loss you may find yourself at a plateau. This lifestyle will allow you to adjust your meals to continue losing weight.
- Coupled with a reasonable exercise routine you will be able to lose more weight while building and toning muscle and still not feel hungry.

- Relief from gastric symptoms

  - High carbohydrate diets are often the culprits if you suffer from heartburn, indigestion and GERD.

  - Symptoms will lessen or disappear altogether when following the ketogenic diet. If you still experience heartburn and reflux, eliminate tomatoes and speak with your physician to determine that your gall bladder is functioning properly.

  - You will find a reduction in gas and bloating as the lower consumption of grains and sugars eliminates the fermentation that occurs in your small intestines.

- Oral health improvements

  - Sugar is known to change the pH of your mouth and causes tooth decay. After a few months following the ketogenic diet you will find that any gingivitis you might be experiencing will decrease or disappear. Check with your dentist for any damage that may remain.

- Increased serotonin and dopamine levels

  ◦ Ketone bodies are known to stabilize your body's neurotransmitters. This will result in fewer mood swings allowing you to feel better about yourself and your life in general.

  ◦ It is unknown at this time whether people taking selective serotonin reuptake inhibitors (SSRIs) will need to continue taking those medications or if they will be able to remove that medicine from their daily routine.

As the lists above show, the unpleasant side effects are temporary and the benefits you will experience by switching to the ketogenic lifestyle are definitely worth the effort.

Chapter 3:

Counting Macros vs. Calories?

If you're picking up this book to learn more about the ketogenic diet then you've probably hear about something called 'macros' or macronutrients. That's what we're going to discuss in this section along with whether or not you should be counting macros or calories. If you get the proportions of macros right, it will make the diet easier to follow where just restricting calories might cause you to fail.

Unfortunately, traditional diets generally don't take into account *what* you are eating, only the calories you are consuming. Portion control can work for a while, but unless you are eating the right foods that will leave you satisfied, eventually your self control will break down. This is what leads to binge eating and giving up on a diet altogether.

If you concentrate on counting your macronutrients rather than the amount of calories you are taking in, you will find yourself eating more of the right foods. This will help you to stick to your diet more easily and you may find that you can allow yourself a few extra grams of carbohydrates if that happens to be one of your absolutely favorite foods.

What Are Macros?

Macros, or macronutrients, are what we consume that provide energy for our cells. There are three necessary for humans; carbohydrates, fats and proteins. Each of these macronutrients provide us with energy when they are broken down. This energy comes in the form of calories.

Each gram of carbohydrates and proteins will be broken down during digestion and provide 4 calories. Fats, however, provide 9 calories for each gram broken down by our systems.

Protein

Protein is associated with building muscle tissue. However it is the main component in all the organs and tissues of your body, hair and enzymes that your body uses on a daily basis. It is made up of amino acids that are necessary for the proper functioning of our bodies but we can make some of them for ourselves. Unfortunately, there are nine amino acids that you must get from the foods we eat. These are called essential amino acids and are found almost exclusively in meats.

Carbohydrates

You can technically survive without carbohydrates but if you cut it out of your diet completely, your body will have to find the small amount of glucose your brain needs from protein. Breaking protein down into glucose actually uses more energy than it provides so a little carbohydrate in your diet is a good thing. Just don't overdo it!

Fats

Fats are often maligned because they are calorie-dense foods. However, they are very important for normal bodily functions. Fats make up the backbone of most of the hormones our body produces, surrounds each nerve to help protect tissues and conduct impulses, and makes our skin and hair healthy and strong.

There are many different kinds of fats that we currently have in our diets; saturated, monounsaturated, polyunsaturated, trans fat, and so many more. The ones you need to be concerned with are Omega-3 and Omega-6 fatty acids. Both are necessary for feeling healthy but Omega-6 fats are much easier to get than the Omega-3. An overdose of Omega-6 fatty acids will result in an increase in inflammation in your joints and muscles. If you're careful of how you balance those two fats, you will feel much better and stay on the track to a more healthy life.

Does Counting Calories on Keto Help?

You may have heard or read that you don't need to count calories when you are following a ketogenic diet. However, that's not *entirely* true. You don't have to count calories while following a ketogenic diet, but doing so can help you get everything you want out of your new lifestyle.

Think of counting calories while on keto as another tool in your arsenal against your weight and to help you get healthy again. There are many websites that will help you determine the number of calories you take in as a matter of course. In order to utilize the ketogenic diet and calorie counting as a dual tool to lose weight, simply reduce the amount of calories taken in by 500 and use the remaining calorie count as your limit. However, you should remember that you don't *need* to take in that many calories.

For example, a 45 year old female weighs 285 pounds, is 5' 7" and has a sedentary lifestyle. She would need to take in roughly 2300 calories to maintain her weight. If she reduced that amount by 500 calories per day to 1800, she would lose approximately 1 pound per week once the initial water weight is gone. However, on the ketogenic diet she may never reach that 1800 calories per day if she eats the right combination of food to keep her feeling full and satisfied. This will translate into higher weight loss per week the farther from that 1800 calorie limit she remains.

The vegetables you eat while on the ketogenic diet will provide you with fiber to feel full longer, the protein and fat will offer you the satiation that keeps you from feeling hungry and you'll experience a higher metabolic rate which will cause you to burn more calories. Because of the sated feeling after eating, you will naturally restrict your caloric intake so that you can lose weight a bit faster than you would on a traditional diet.

Weight Loss & Muscle Building

Most people who begin following a ketogenic lifestyle will not be those who are already fairly fit and have a lot of muscles already. However, that doesn't mean that you might not get to that point once you have gotten close to your ideal weight and your desired health level.

Once your body is fully adapted to this new diet and you have lost as much weight as necessary to feel more energized you will be able to adjust your menus to accommodate building strength and muscle as well. When you reach the point in the 'standard' ketogenic diet where you feel like building and toning muscle is right for you, you will be able to alter the diet to what is called 'targeted' or 'cyclical'. Both of those versions of the ketogenic diet allow more carbohydrate consumption so that you can take in enough glucose to feed your muscles without knocking yourself out of ketosis.

The targeted ketogenic diet allows you to take in extra carbohydrates around your exercise times. This diet is a compromise between the standard ketogenic diet which we have been discussing and the cyclical ketogenic diet that will be described in a few moments. This form of the diet allows you to perform a high intensity workout without falling out of ketosis for a long period of time. The intake of more carbohydrates before a workout is beneficial because you will have the glucose necessary for your muscles to work but all that extra glucose is burned off during your workout so your metabolism isn't altered for more than the 30 minutes or so that your workout takes. The TKD is for beginner or intermittent exercisers because it allows a slight increase in carbohydrate intake but keeps you in ketosis without a shock to your system.

The cyclical ketogenic diet is for more advanced athletic trainers and bodybuilders. This form is used for maximum muscle building. However, you may end up gaining some body fat. This is because it is easy to overeat on this form of the diet despite the extremely depleting workouts you will be doing on this diet. The CKD tends to have you following the standard ketogenic diet for 5 or 6 days followed by 1 or 2 days of high carbohydrate eating. The reason this doesn't work for beginners is that it can take up to 3 weeks for your body to go fully into ketosis. The goal of this form of the lifestyle is to temporarily switch out of ketosis in order to refill the amount of glycogen in the muscles to support the intense workout during your next cycle. Remember, if you choose to do this sort of diet, that you must completely deplete the amount of glycogen during your training session. The intensity of your training will depend on the amount of carbohydrates to took in during your carbo-loading phase.

Is it Possible Not to Lose Weight on a Ketogenic Diet?

This isn't just a plateau where you have been losing weight but the losses have tapered off or stopped altogether for a week or so. This is in case where you are actually not losing weight and finding it difficult to get into ketosis OR you've been following it and something has happened to make it hard for you to keep to your new lifestyle. These things can be stress, the holidays, or even a stretch of time where you were invited out more than once a week.

The short answer to this question is **yes**, it is possible that you will experience a lack of weight-loss while on a ketogenic diet. However, there are several reasons behind this and most of them can be dealt with by making some adjustments to your menu plan and lifestyle.

- *You may be eating too many carbohydrates.*

  ○ Decrease your carb intake.

  ○ Increase the amount of coconut oil in your diet. Coconut oil is a medium chain triglyceride and is more easily digestible and used for immediate energy needs.

- *You may be eating too much or too little protein.*

  ○ Protein is a very satisfying macronutrient.

  ○ Eating too little protein will lead to muscle loss.

  ○ Eating too much protein will lead to an increase in glycogen in your cells which will kick you out of ketosis.

- *Cheating on carbs.*

  ◦ You need to be very disciplined and count every single carb that you eat.

  ◦ Anti-caking agents are used in many spices, table salt and other baking items like baking powder, baking soda and cocoa. Other food additives like emulsifiers/stabilizers, thickeners and gelling agents are also often carbohydrate based.

  ◦ If you find yourself nibbling here and there, you will need to determine if you are actually hungry or if it is out of habit.

- *You may be eating too many fats.*

  ◦ Yes, it's a high fat diet. However, that doesn't mean you can eat 5000 calories worth of fats and expect to lose weight.

  ◦ Calories aren't **as big** a deal in the ketogenic diet so long as you are getting the correct amounts of *all* the macronutrients, but do be aware of how much you are taking in.
  ◦ You may be consuming the wrong kinds of fats as well. Be sure to take in only beneficial fats while on the ketogenic diet.

- *You may be taking in too many artificial sweeteners.*

  ○ Be aware that any ketogenic recipe may call for Stevia or Erythritol for sweetening. These can cause cravings which can make you stop losing weight.

  ○ Artificial sweeteners often contain anti-caking agents which add to your carbohydrate intake. These are easy to miss.
  ○ Chewing gum, mints, cough syrups and other food items or medications can contain artificial sweeteners and should be avoided whenever possible.

- *Excessive dairy and nuts.*

  ○ Milk is seldom included in a ketogenic diet plan because it contains high amounts of lactose which will be transformed directly into glucose during digestion.
  ○ Limit your cheese and yogurt intake to reduce the amount of dairy you are consuming.

  ○ Nuts are often included in a ketogenic diet but always in limited amounts due to the high caloric content.
  ○ Too much dairy and nuts can kick you out of ketosis because they are calorie-dense foods and are very easy to overindulge.

- *You may be close to your target weight.*

  ○ Losing weight becomes more difficult the closer you get to your ideal weight.

  ○ To continue losing weight once you have reached this level, you may need to adjust your macronutrient intake or increase your exercise intensity, or both.

- *You may be under more stress than you think.*

  ○ When you are stressed your body will produce more cortisol which is what makes your body store fat and make losing weight more difficult.

  ○ Stress is also linked to hypothyroidism as well as adrenal issues that can effect your metabolism.

  ○ Gentle exercise and sunshine will help to ease the amount of stress you are under. If you feel yourself becoming stressed, go for a walk outside for about 20 minutes and you will find yourself feeling better and the desire to stress-eat will disappear.

- *Your circadian rhythms may be disrupted.*

  ○ Sleep is essential for long-term weight loss.

  ○ Try to sleep before midnight and get between 7 and 9 hours of sleep each night.

- Unless you find yourself ravenous when you wake in the morning, try to avoid eating in the 3 hours before you go to sleep. If you must have a bedtime snack, make sure it has a balance of fats, protein and carbs so that you won't fall out of ketosis.

- *You might be exercising too much.*

  - Too much exercise can be as bad for you as not enough when you are in the losing weight phase.

  - Remember that muscle weighs more than fat so even if you are following your diet strictly and still not losing weight, this may be the reason. This should only occur if you are past the losing weight phase and moving into the muscle toning and building phase.

  - Adjust your macro intake to accommodate your exercise routine.

- *You might have a thyroid or adrenal issue that you have never been diagnosed with or been tested for.*

  - Consult with your physician for testing to be certain you are not dealing with a thyroid or adrenal dysfunction.
  - Low-carbohydrate diets are not suggested for anyone with hypothyroidism or adrenal disease.

- *You may be experiencing a lack of leptin production.*

  ○ Leptin is a hormone put off by fat cells that tells the body to stop eating.

  ○ Elevated leptin levels indicates satiety after eating.

  ○ As you lose weight you will have fewer fat cells so your body may not have high enough leptin levels to signal satiety.

  ○ This can be remedied by eating foods rich in both fat and protein.

- *You may be using artificial sweeteners that contain sugar alcohols.*

  ○ Sweeteners such as Stevia, Swerve, erythritol and chicory root do not contain sugar alcohols so are better for use in a ketogenic recipe.

  ○ Products labeled as 'low-fat' are often full of added sugars. The reason behind this is that something must be added to make it taste good since fat is what carries flavor. If fat is taken out of a food product, something else must be used to carry the flavor and the secondary carrier is a carbohydrate.

- You may not be getting enough water and electrolytes.

  ◦ Water is vital for fat loss so you need to make sure you are properly hydrated.

  ◦ Water suppresses the appetite and helps you metabolize fat.

  ◦ Proper intake of electrolytes such as magnesium, potassium and sodium help to keep you from retaining water as well as making sure that your muscles work properly.

  ◦ The right amount of electrolytes will also keep your muscles from cramping. The toxins built up by cramps can cause cravings for both salt and carbohydrates because of the inflammation surrounding the cramped muscles.

What Can I Do If I Plateau?

Plateauing is not altogether unexpected on the ketogenic diet. It happens in any kind of diet that you might choose to follow.

When you lose weight, your metabolism will decline. This causes you to burn fewer calories than you did at your heavier weight. The slower your metabolism, the slower you will lose weight even if you eat the same number of calories that had originally helped you lose weight. When the calories you burn equals the number of calories you eat, you will reach a plateau.

There are a few ways that you can break through a plateau so that you can continue losing weight until you are ready to begin a gentle exercise and muscle toning routine.

- *Eat more fiber.*

  ○ You can add psyllium husk to nearly any food. It is used as a thickener as well as to make ketogenic bread.

  ○ Additional fiber will help you feel full longer and will help to reduce the amount of food you are eating.

- *Figure out your attitude toward food.* Knowing what motivates you to eat will help you to create your plan to overcome those unproductive tendencies.

  ○ If you are anxious, nervous or depressed, you might find that you eat to feel better. This is called emotional hunger.

    ▪ Emotional hunger comes on suddenly. It is often overwhelming and feels urgent, possibly painful.
    ▪ Emotional hunger makes you crave specific foods, especially comfort foods. Unfortunately, those cravings are often for sugary or fatty foods. Fatty foods on the ketogenic diet are not always bad for you but when it is emotionally driven the fatty foods you might crave aren't necessarily the beneficial fats encouraged on your keto diet.
    ▪ Emotional hunger isn't satisfied when your stomach is full. You will often find yourself uncomfortably full which will lead to indigestion, heartburn, sour stomach, diarrhea or constipation and sometimes vomiting.

- Emotional hunger doesn't come from your stomach since you are craving something based upon the texture, the taste or the smell of the food.
- If you are prone to emotional hunger, you will often feel guilty because you know that you are not eating for nutritional reasons. Regret and shame are also part of the emotions that occur after emotional eating which can lead to continued emotional eating.

- Emotional hunger is the most difficult to overcome but it is still possible. Remember that

most emotional eating is caused by unpleasant feelings but it can also be used as a reward for an accomplishment or when celebrating a holiday. You can do any of the following to get out of the habit of eating when your emotions are involved.

- Identify your trigger. Are you stressed? Are you stuffing or silencing uncomfortable emotions? Are you bored or overly tired? Is it a habit from childhood to reward yourself for something you've done? Do you feel nervous when you're out with friends?

Distract yourself when you find yourself wanting to eat emotionally. Call a friend or family member. Walk your dog or play with your cat. Expend nervous energy by dancing to

- your favorite song or taking a brisk walk. Enjoy a cup of tea or glass of wine in a hot bath with soothing oils. Read a book, explore outside, work on a hobby you enjoy.

- Take 30 minutes for yourself every day. Exercise. Meditate. If you are religious, read your holy book and pray. Take a nap. Spend time with people who enhance your life.

  ○ If you are impulsive you may need to remove temptations from your house and take someone with you when you go grocery shopping to tell you 'no' when you get to the checkout counter.

  ○ If you don't pay attention to what you eat then you will want to avoid situations where food is available while you are doing something else such as watching TV.
  ○ Engage in fasting and high intensity exercise once in a while.

Intermittent Exercise & Fasting

High intensity and intermittent exercise and fasting can help to break a plateau and get you back on the weight loss track. Fasting once in a while is good to help to cleanse your body of built up toxins and to jump start your metabolism when it gets to the point of plateauing. Intermittent high intensity exercise can also jump start your metabolism by improving your glucose tolerance and burning excess calories. Because of the intensity any glycol that remains built up in the muscles will be depleted which will help you to remain in ketosis. Since glycol requires water to be stored then you will have more water-weight that will be lost as well.

- *Intermittent High Intensity Exercise*

  ○ Also known as interval training.

  ○ This is an exercise technique where you alternate intense anaerobic exercise with short recovery periods.
  ○ One effect is that you will burn more calories in less time compared to low intensity workouts which are generally aerobic exercises.
  ○ 15-20 minute workouts with a 5 minute warm up and a 5 minute cool down to avoid cramping.

  ○ The idea behind anaerobic exercise is to cause your muscles to feel fatigued in a very short period of time. Below are some suggested exercises that will accomplish this within that 10 minute period of intense exercise.

    · **Heavy weight lifting.** You should only be able to lift this weight 3 to 6 times before your muscles feel fatigued.
    · **High speed burpees.** These should be performed as quickly as possible so that they are anaerobic rather than aerobic. To perform a burpee follow the directions below.

      ▪ Stand with your hands at your sides.

      ▪ Squat down and place your hands on the floor about shoulder width apart.

      Jump your feet back so that you are in the push up position.

■

- Perform a push up.

- Jump your feet back to your hands so you are squatted again.

- Leap into the air.

- Land with your knees bent and repeat.

- See how many you can perform in 60 seconds and rest for 60 seconds between repetitions. Continue until your muscles feel fatigued or 10 minutes.

- If the push up or the leap are too strenuous, you can omit those until you are better able to accomplish them.

- **Sprinting.**

  - This requires an all-out effort which makes it anaerobic.

  - If you don't have access to a track or other flat area to run, you can do sprints-in-place.

    ○ Start by jogging in place to get your rhythm.

- Lift your knees so that your thighs are parallel to the floor. Pump your arms vigorously.
- Pick up the pace until you are going as fast as you can.

- Continue for 30 to 60 seconds.

- Rest for 60 seconds and repeat for remaining time.

- **Double-under Jump Rope**

  - This is a high-intensity jump rope exercise that is an effective workout often used by boxers.

  - Start by jumping rope normally to get used to the movement.

  - When you feel ready, jump a little higher and increase the speed you are turning the rope.

  - Continue jumping rope normally until you are ready to do another double-under.

  - Once you have perfected your technique at this exercise, you can begin to do multiple double-unders back to back.

  - If you are just beginning double-unders, jump rope with intermittent double-unders for 3 minutes. Rest for 30 seconds

■ before performing a second 3 minute set.

■ If you are competent at double-unders, perform 10 in a row, rest 30 seconds, perform 20 in a row, rest 30 seconds, and then perform 30 in a row with 30 second rest periods until your exercise time limit is up.

- **Kettle bell swings**

  ■ You can perform this exercise using a single dumbbell or a heavy weight in a bag that won't tear.

  ■ This exercise targets hamstrings, lower back, upper back and glutes.

  ■ In order to perform this exercise, follow the directions below.

  ○ Hold the weight in both hands in front of your hips.

  ○ Bend your knees slightly and push your butt backwards to lower the weight to hang between your knees.
  ○ Shove your hips forward and use that momentum to swing the weight upward to shoulder height. Keep your arms straight but control the weight to keep it from swinging too far.

44

- ◦ Let the weight swing back to knee height and repeat.

- ◦ Try to do 15 swings per minutes.

- ◦ Do not allow your back to round as this can cause lower back injury.

- *Intermittent Fasting*

  ◦ This is exactly as it sounds. You will fast between 14 and 36 hours with a very strict 'feeding window'. For the longer fast periods, you can split your 'window' in two if necessary.

  - ▪ If you fast for 14 hours, your 'feeding window' is 2-3 hours.

  - ▪ If you fast for 24 hours, your 'feeding window' is 4-6 hours.

  - ▪ If you fast for 36 hours, your 'feeding window' is 6-8 hours.

  ◦ The idea is that you will be eating as much as you want during your 'feeding window' but when you are in your 'fasting period' you will not take in anything with caloric value.
  - ▪ **Feeding Window**

      - ▪ Try to reach your macronutrient target without restricting yourself but make sure you only eat to satiety.

      - It may not be possible to reach your macronutrient

- target and that is perfectly acceptable.

  ◦ Eat all of your protein. Remember that if you eat less protein than required, you may lose muscles, decrease your metabolic rate and end up burning less body fat.
  ◦ Eat as much of your fats as necessary to become satisfied.

  ◦ Carbohydrates are the least important to consume during this feeding window. If you choose to include carbohydrates, then keep your intake to less than 20 grams.

- **Fasting Window**

  - When fasting, you will only consume liquids with zero caloric and/or nutritional value.

  - Water is obviously allowed.

  - Black coffee or tea sweetened with Stevia or erythritol are allowed.

While neither High Intensity Intermittent Exercise and Intermittent Fasting are optimal for weight loss, they are both good tools to use to break through a stubborn plateau. Once you have gotten back to losing weight you can adjust your macronutrient and caloric intake so that you can continue to lose weight. At this point, you should be close to where you can begin gentle, aerobic exercises to tone and build lean muscle mass.

Chapter 4:

Okay Foods, Meal Plans & Other Important Information

T his section will give you a lot of basic information that may seem a bit overwhelming. Don't let it discourage you when you see many foods on the 'absolutely avoid' list, especially if they are some of your favorites. You really can make this work for you.

Do You Need Any Special Equipment?

While you don't necessarily **need** any special equipment, there are a few kitchen appliances and tools that will make it easier to follow a ketogenic recipe.

> A high-power blender, such as a Vita-Mix, will help because it makes pureeing foods for sauces extremely simple. With such a blender you won't
> • need to worry about partially cooking hard root vegetables before pureeing them.

- A food processor with a shredding/grating blade is always helpful. Otherwise you'll be in danger of skinning your knuckles or taking off your fingernails on those dreaded box graters.

- A mandolin is a very useful kitchen implement. It will allow you to slice, ribbon and julienne your vegetables in a much shorter time than if you had to use a knife for those tasks.

- A vegetable spiralizer, or a Veggeti Slicer, is handy for making vegetable 'spaghetti' for some of your recipes. Different textures of the foods incorporated into many ketogenic meals make them more fun and appetizing.

- A juicer might be a helpful appliance as well. Sometimes it's just easier to get your meals in liquid form and a juicer can make it that much easier. Though if you have a Vita-Mix blender, a juicer might not be necessary.

An immersion blender may not be necessary if you have a food processor or a Vita-Mix blender. However, it is useful for when you don't want to have to transfer hot liquid that you need to liquefy or puree into the blender or food processor. It is also useful for when you are making smaller amounts. A digital kitchen scale is very useful if the aim of following the ketogenic diet is to lose weight. Measuring cups are not the same in all countries and can vary from maker to maker. It is always better to

- measure by weight for most foods. A slightly wrong amount can ruin your recipe and add extra carbohydrates for which you haven't accounted.

- A steamer or a basket that allows you to steam in a dutch oven that you might already have isn't essential but it is useful to have. Steaming is the most gentle way to cook some tougher vegetables without losing many nutrients.

- A citrus juicer isn't necessary but since you will often need fresh squeezed lemon or lime juice for many ketogenic recipes, it is a good item to have in your kitchen.

- A zester will also find a lot of use when following the ketogenic diet since many of the recipes call for lemon, lime or orange zest as well as the juice.

- A food saver or some other vacuum sealing unit allows you to keep your foods fresher longer. You can chop vegetables for your recipes ahead of time, seal them and refrigerate or freeze them for later use. You can marinate your meats prior to cooking or even store your leftovers for additional meals.

What Foods Can You Eat?

Fats

- Avocado Oil

- Almond Oil

- Beef Tallow; should be from grass fed cattle

- Butter; organic if possible

- Chicken Fat

- Duck Fat

- Ghee; goat butter with the milk solids removed

- Lard; NOT hydrogenated, organic if possible

- Macadamia Oil

- Mayonnaise; read the label to be sure it has no carbs in it

- Olive Oil

- Sesame Oil

-

- Flaxseed Oil

- Hemp Oil

- Coconut Oil

- Coconut Butter

- Coconut Cream; concentrated, organic

Proteins

- Beef

- Lamb

- Veal

- Goat

- Wild game

- Pork; read the label of ham, sausage and bacon to avoid
- added sugar Chicken

- Turkey

- Duck

- Goose

- Game birds

- Anchovies

- Calamari

- Catfish

- Cod

- Flounder

- Halibut

- Herring

- Mackerel

- Mahi-mahi

Salmon; canned is allowed, read the label for added sugar or carb-fillers Sardines

-
-
- Scrod

- Sole

- Snapper

- Trout

- Tuna; canned is allowed, read the label for added sugar or carb-fillers Clams
-

- Crab

- Lobster

- Scallops

- Shrimp

- Squid

- Mussels

- Oysters

- Whole eggs; cooked in a variety of ways

- Peanut Butter; read the label for carbohydrates, natural is best Tempeh; read the label for carbohydrates

- Tofu; read the label for carbohydrates

- Edamame; read the label for carbohydrates

- Whey protein powders; be very careful about the contents of the product, determine the amount of added sugars and fillers that may be included

Vegetables

- Alfalfa sprouts

- Asparagus

- Avocado; Hass is best for eating

- Bamboo shoots

- Bean sprouts

- Beet greens

-
- Bell peppers *
- Bok choy
- Broccoli
- Brussels sprouts
- Cabbage
- Carrots *
- Cauliflower
- Celery
- Celery root
- Chard
- Chives
- Collard greens
- Cucumbers
- Dandelion greens

- Pickles; dill

- Garlic

- Kale

- Leeks

- Arugula

- Boston butter lettuce

- Chicory

- Endive

- Escarole

- Fennel

- Radicchio

- Romaine

- Mushrooms

- Olives

Onions *

- Radishes

- Sauerkraut; be careful of added sugar unless making it yourself

- Scallions

- Shallots

- Snow peas

- Spinach

- Summer squash *

- Tomatoes *

- Turnips

- Zucchini

- Water chestnuts

* These vegetables are higher in carbohydrates so intake should be limited.

Dairy Products

- Heavy whipping cream

- Sour cream; full fat, read labels for additives and fillers

- Cottage cheese; full fat

- Cheddar

- Swiss

- Colby

- Monterey Jack

- Provolone

- Munster

- Gouda

- Farmer cheese

- Blue cheese

- Cream cheese

- Marscapone

- Yogurt; unsweetened, full fat, Greek, limit how much you eat due to the higher carb content

Nuts & Seeds

It is best to soak and/or roast nuts and seeds to get rid of any possible anti-nutrients they may contain. Since they are very high in carbs you will need to limit your intake. Too many nuts and seeds can cause increased inflammation so you should not depend upon them for all of your protein needs. Nuts and seeds can also cause a disruption in you moods.

- Macadamias

- Pecans

- Almonds

- Walnuts

- Cashews

- Pistachios

- Chestnuts

- Almond flour

- Peanuts

- Pumpkin seeds

- Sunflower seeds

- Sesame seeds

- Hemp seeds

- Chia seeds

Beverages

All beverages should be unsweetened. Use artificial sweeteners sparingly. Be certain that all beverages are decaffeinated since caffeine can increase blood sugar.

- Bone broth

- Decaffeinated coffee

- Decaffeinated tea

- Herbal tea

- Water

- Flavored seltzer water

- Lemon juice

- Lime juice

- Almond milk

- Hazelnut milk

- Cashew milk

- Coconut milk

- Soy milk

- Hemp milk

Fruits, Spices & Miscellaneous

Most fruits should be avoided since they are high in carbohydrates in the form of fructose. However, there are some berries that can be enjoyed in small amounts once in a while.

- Blueberries

- Strawberries

- Raspberries

- Cranberries

- Blackberries

Any spice that you do not grind yourself will contain carbohydrates. Commercially made spice mixes usually contain added sugar. For salting dishes, you should use sea salt rather than regular iodized salt which is often combined with powdered dextrose to prevent clumping. However, there are some spices that have negligible amounts of carbs added that you will find in many ketogenic recipes. Despite those carbs being negligible doesn't mean you shouldn't count them. There are websites that allow you to put in your complete recipe, including spices, and the site will calculate all of your macros as well as calories which will help you include those 'negligible' carbs.

- Black pepper

- Basil

- Cayenne pepper

Chili powder

-
- Cilantro

- Cinnamon

- Cumin

- Ginger

- Cardamom

- Bay leaves

- Oregano

- Parsley

- Rosemary

- Sage

- Thyme

- Turmeric

Other items you can enjoy in limited amounts are Japanese Shirataki noodles, pork rinds and 85-90% chocolate.

Pork rinds are a good substitute for bread crumbs but they are high in protein so you should limit your use of them.

Some ketogenic recipes, especially desserts, require some form of sweetening and you really should be careful about how much artificial sweetener you use since you are trying to get a more natural diet going. That being said, the best sweeteners to use are natural like honey or agave. You just need to be very careful about how much you use and follow the recipe exactly so that you are not adding too many carbohydrates to your daily allotment.

Foods You Should Absolutely Avoid

Sugars & Sweeteners

- Maple syrup

- Malt syrup

- Treacle

- Carob syrup

- Brown sugar

- Turbinado sugar

- White sugar

- Confectioner's or powdered sugar

- Beet sugar

- Cane juice

- Cane syrup

- Caramel

- Panela

- Panocha

- Coconut sugar

- Date sugar

- Corn syrup

- Sorghum

- Molasses

- Rice syrup

- Maltose

- Barley malt

- Maltodextrin

- Fruit syrups

- Fruit juice concentrate

- Tapioca syrup

- And any food or food additive that ends in -ose.

Grains & Grain Products

- Wheat

- Barley

- Oats

- Rye

- Sorghum

- Tricale

- Spelt

- Rice

- Bread

- Muffins

- Rolls

- Bread crumbs

- Waffles

- Pancakes

- Pasta

- Any commercial cereals; hot and cold

- Tortillas

- Crackers

- Cookies

- Tarts

- Cakes
- Pies

- Pretzels

- Oatmeal

- Cous Cous

- Cream of wheat

- Quinoa

- Kashi

- Cornbread

- Tamale wrappers

- Corn chips

- Grits

- Polenta

- Popcorn

- Cornmeal

Fruits, Vegetables & Legumes

- Apples

- Bananas

- Plantains

- Pears

- Oranges

- Grapefruits

- Peaches

- Apricots

- Currents

- Cantaloupe

- Honeydew Melon

- Watermelon

- Cherries

- Dates

- Figs

- Gooseberries

- Grapes

- Raisins

- Guava

- Mango

- Nectarines

- Kiwi

- Papaya

- Plums

- Pineapple

- Pumpkin

- Pomegranates

- Potatoes

- Sweet potatoes

- Hash browns

- Potato chips

- Tater tots

- French fries

- Mashed potatoes

- Corn

- Lima beans

- Peas

- Okra

- Artichokes

- Kidney beans

- Black beans

- Black-eyed peas

- Chickpeas

- Great northern beans

- Vegetable juice concentrate

- Lentils

Other Foods You Should Avoid

- Canned soups

- Canned stews

- Processed, boxed 'convenience' foods

- Foods listed as 'low-fat', 'low-carb', 'sugar-free', etc. This includes prepared foods and snack bars produced for known HFLC diets like Atkins and South Beach. The reason is that the preservatives tend to be carbohydrate based which can mitigate the benefits of going low-carb.

- Beer

- Hard liquor

Sweet or dessert wines; dry wines are allowed in

- limited amounts Carbonated beverages (aka Soda-pop); both diet and non-diet

- Milk; liquid milk contains lactose. Cheese and yogurt is allowed since the fermentation process reduces the amount of lactose in the milk solids.

Chapter 5:

How Can You Make This Work For You?

Many people want to follow a ketogenic diet. You may know that it is the lifestyle for you but you're not sure if you can make it work with your busy schedule. You don't have to be a stay-at-home parent or spend all your time in the kitchen just to make the meals either.

With the ketogenic diet you will decide what kind of foods you'll eat and with the internet having hundreds of sites that have recipes for this lifestyle, it should be no problem at all to find meals you can fix and enjoy in a short period of time.

It doesn't matter if you are the CEO of a Fortune 500 company or a Kindergarten teacher. If you need to make this change, you will find a way to make it work. The lifestyle may not be for everyone, but it should be.

Determining Your Numbers and Cooking For One

The key to understanding the ketogenic lifestyle and making it work for you by cooking your own food is to remember that you are switching out the carbohydrates in your diet for a higher fat and more moderate protein intake.

Fats have very limited effect on blood sugar levels and insulin production in your body. However, protein does affect both of those if you eat more than your body requires. The recommended amount of protein that should be consumed is 0.36 grams per pound. Unfortunately, the common diet today suggests much higher amounts than you actually need so all that extra protein that is not broken down to the 9 essential amino acids will become glucose which is stored as fat. This higher level of glucose will boost the insulin levels in your blood which will stall the body's ability to release and burn ketones.

The ketogenic diet plan works best when you track the amount of carbs you eat. All ketogenic plans allows a fairly broad range of grams per day of carbohydrates, between 20 and 60 grams per day. However, it is suggested that if you are just beginning the new lifestyle you should limit your carbohydrate intake to no more than 20 grams per day.

The amount of protein you will consume will not be based upon your current weight but on the weight you want to reach. Just because a person weighs 350 pounds, that doesn't mean they will be eating 120 or more grams of protein. Your protein intake will be based upon your ideal weight as well as your gender and how much you exercise. Remember than men require slightly more protein than women. Those who have a moderately active exercise routine also require more protein than those who lead a more sedentary life.

So how do you determine your percentages and the grams of each macronutrient you need to consume on the ketogenic diet? Let's work with a couple examples so that you can determine the numbers for yourself.

EX 1. Mary is a 40 year old woman, 5' 7", 285 pounds and is a receptionist who does not exercise on a weekly basis. Her ideal weight is roughly between 120-160 pounds. She chooses to reach the highest end of her ideal weight when starting the ketogenic diet; 160 pounds.

Protein: 160 X 0.36 = 57.6 grams per day

Mary's intake of protein each day will be rounded up to 58 grams which will be set at 20% protein consumption. This will give her the proper amount of essential amino acids her body needs to function properly without increasing her blood glucose and insulin levels. Once she has her required grams of protein, she will be able to determine her carbohydrate percentage. Let's say that Mary chooses 5% as her carb intake.

Carbohydrate: 58 / 4 = 14.5 grams per day

Mary will round up again to give her 15 grams of carbohydrates per day. Eliminating all grains, most fruits and starchy vegetables will allow her to eat plenty of vegetables and still maintain this minimal intake of carbohydrates.

Now Mary needs to figure out the amount of fats she will consume. It's a bit easier since the remaining 75% of her diet will consist of nutritious and healthy fats, but she still needs to know the grams so that she doesn't overdo and make the ketogenic diet not work properly for her.

Fats: $(58 \times 3) + (15 \times 3) = 219$ grams per day

So this is Mary's ketogenic 75:20:5 intake; 219 grams of fats, 58 grams of protein and 15 grams of carbohydrates.

This is one way for Mary to determine how much she needs to eat each day.

EX 2. Mary's doctor is willing to allow her to try this diet and will keep a close watch on her health. However, he has suggested that she combine calorie counting along with the ketogenic plan. Mary and her doctor have decided that a 1500 calorie diet would allow her to lose weight and still not be hungry while living the ketogenic lifestyle.

Fats: $1500 \times 0.75 = 1125$ calories from fat

1125 cal / 9 cal per gram = 125 grams per day

This may seem like a lot of fat to eat per day but you won't be resorting to eating sticks of butter. 1 tablespoon of butter has 11 grams of fat so if you add olive oil, avocados and coconut oil as they appear in your recipes then it won't seem as if you are eating quite that much on a daily basis.

Protein:

1500 X 0.20 = 300 calories from protein

300 / 4 = 75 grams per day

Yes, this amount is more than what was found using the recommended amount per pound of ideal body weight but this will still keep her from losing muscle mass and give her all the amino acids she needs.

Carbohydrate:

1500 X 0.05 = 75 calories from carbs

75 / 4 = 18.75 grams per day

This amount too is slightly more than when using a pure percentage calculation, but Mary has the option of reducing this amount as well if she chooses.

Both of the previous examples will allow Mary to lose weight and begin feeling better. As she slims down and her health returns, the energy this lifestyle offers her will give her the chance to increase her exercise routine.

Whenever you find yourself plateauing while following this lifestyle exactly it is usually an indication that you need to alter your percentages. You may need to increase your protein and exercise routine, which won't be a problem once you start feeling more healthy. If you are increasing your protein you will need to decrease your carbohydrate intake as well. The amount of healthy fats you take in on a daily basis should remain the same with only slight fluctuations as you alter your routines.

If you are also counting calories while following this lifestyle you will need to reduce your caloric intake to continue losing weight if you plateau and have not reached your chosen weight. Simple re-calculate your grams per day with the new calorie amount and adjust your meal plan as needed.

Finding Meal Plans That Fit Your Life

Finding a meal plan that will fit your life is easy to do in the day and age of the internet. Websites abound with ready made meal plans and hundreds of thousands of recipes that can be used with the ketogenic diet.

You have your percentages and the recommended grams you should consume each day so now there are a few things that you need to consider and do so that you are successful with this lifestyle.

> **Get a carbohydrate counter guide.** This is a list of how many carbohydrates are in every single food that you might encounter during your new lifestyle. It also

covers all of the highly processed foods that you were eating before choosing to go keto. Keeping track of your carbs is the essential part of this program so a carb counter will help you know and understand how to do it correctly.

Do a carb sweep. Go through your kitchen and food storage areas. Get rid of all your high carb foods, processed snack foods and any 'complex carbs'. This includes anything advertised as 'low carb' since those products can contain hidden carbs that will throw you out of ketosis.

Go shopping. You will want to restock your pantry and refrigerator with foods that are going to fit your new lifestyle and help you avoid temptation. With this new lifestyle you will find yourself shopping more often. Since many vegetables only last for about a week, you'll want to be sure that you use the freshest possible produce in your recipes.

Think about what you will be eating and how to plan your meals. This helps you when you go to the grocery store. If you know exactly what you're going to be having for the week, you will be less likely to simply wander and pick up whatever looks good.

Change your morning routine. If you stop at the coffee shop on the way to work and pick up a bagel with

- your coffee, make your coffee at home and enjoy it with a couple of fried eggs instead.

- **Drink plenty of water.** As you stop taking in carbohydrates your body will start getting rid of excess water as your glycogen levels decrease. This can lead to dehydration. You may also need to drink electrolyte replacement drinks but be sure to count the carb amounts since most sports drinks have added sweeteners. Otherwise you can simply add salt to your meals and take magnesium and potassium supplements.

- **Consider taking natural supplements.** These help support cellular respiration and reduces inflammation by increasing your antioxidant levels.

  - Alpha-lipoic acid – 200-600 mg per day

  - L-glutamine – 500-1000 mg per day

  - CoQ10 – 100-300 mg per day

  - Magnesium citrate or Malate – 400-600 mg per day

  - Potassium – 99 mg per day

  - Vitamin C – 500 mg per day

- Vitamin D – 400-2500 IU per day

- Vitamin E – 100 mg per day

- L-carnitine – 500-1000 mg per day

- A multi-vitamin without iron will give you all the B vitamins you need in addition to what you ingest with each meal.
- Iron is not recommended since bacteria and viruses will use any extra to find a foothold in your intestines to make you ill. Small amounts are necessary and can be found in red meats and some leafy green vegetables but excess amounts can be dangerous.

Purchase Ketostix Reagent Strips. These are used to check your ketone levels so that you can be sure that you are in nutritional ketosis. You should be able to find either the urine or blood strips in your pharmacy. If you are using the blood ketone strips you will need a special meter which can also be found in your pharmacy.

Keep track of your daily food intake. Keep a journal or spreadsheet that includes the amount of food you eat, the macronutrient gram amounts as well as your calories if you are counting those. This will allow

- you to track how the diet makes you feel. You can look back and see what works for you.

Don't beat yourself up for 'cheating'. Not everyone will be following the ketogenic diet. You will encounter your 'old' foods at workplace parties, at get togethers with friends and family or at the holidays. So long as you don't scarf down a baked potato or a plate of chili-cheese fries along with that beer you will be fine. You can minimize the possibility of dropping out of ketosis even at these events by eating the parts that you *know* fit with your diet; salad, meat, cheeses. A few extra grams of carbohydrates *once* won't disrupt your

- new lifestyle all that much. You may need to do 'damage control' the next day to get yourself back on track but just because you are following the ketogenic lifestyle, it doesn't mean you have to become a hermit to do so.

Throw out your bathroom scale. Seriously, get rid of it. Hide it at the very least. Even if you started a ketogenic diet to lose weight, you don't need to *focus* on your weight. Your weight will vary between 1 and 5 pounds every day and weighing yourself every day without seeing the numbers go down will make you crazy! Instead, focus on the way you feel and how your clothes are fitting. So long as your health is improving and your clothes are getting looser, you are doing everything right and the new lifestyle is working.

So long as you choose recipes that will follow the percentages of fats, proteins and carbohydrates, you will find it very easy to fit ketogenics into your busy life routine. If you find that you are running into very similar recipes by doing an internet search on ketogenic recipes, you can always utilize recipes from the very similar Paleo diet. If you choose to use paleo recipes you will need to run the recipes through a carb counter to be sure that you are not taking in too many. The best use of paleo recipes is to alter them into a keto diet recipe which is fairly easy to do.

In the next chapter you will find some sample recipes that will show you what to look for in a recipe. You may also get some ideas for altering meals that you and your family already enjoy so that they are more ketogenic friendly.

You Can Enjoy Snacks & Even Dine Out!

While most people on the ketogenic diet find that they do perfectly fine on 2 or 3 meals each day, others find that they do need snacks to maintain that balance between ketosis and not feeling hunger. This often happens when your routine is interrupted from your regular schedule. If that is the case, you can often have a few things on hand to curb that hunger until you can get home where you can eat your regular meal. You just need to be sure that you are counting the macros included in your snack into your daily intake. Below is a short list of items that make a good snack for when you need a little extra boost to your day.

- Cheese – about 2 ounces of mozzarella, cheddar, co-jack in slice or stick form. Be sure to check the label for carbohydrates as well as the fat and protein.

- Sliced ham and cream cheese roll-ups.

- Olives

- Nuts

- A boiled egg

- Canned sardines in olive oil or sauce. Again, be certain to check the label for how many grams of carbs, proteins and fats you're adding to your diet and compensate for them.

- Leftover meat from a previous meal

- Boiled or steamed shrimp

- Smoked salmon strips spread with cream cheese

- ½ Haas avocado and half a medium tomato cubed and tossed with mayonnaise Beef jerky cured without sugar

- Tuna salad spread on cucumber rounds

If you find that you are always getting hungry between meals you may not be eating enough fat and possibly protein as well. You shouldn't be afraid of fat. Increase the amount of beneficial fats so that you can remain satisfied and no longer need the between meal snacks.

Another time that you may feel the ketogenic diet is inconvenient is when you are invited out to eat with your friends or must attend dinners for business. You shouldn't have any difficulty at restaurants since you can request that the potato, fries or rice be switched for a salad or steamed vegetables. You can ask for extra butter to spread onto your steak or vegetables which will lend extra flavor and add moisture.

If you are simply going out with your friends to a fast food joint or a sports bar to watch the game, hamburgers or chicken wings are often the least bad option even with the sauces that come on the wings. It is obvious that you should avoid the soft drinks and fries. You can always drink water even if your friends are indulging in a beer or three, be the designated driver so everyone gets home safely. Pizza toppings are okay and the stricter you are with yourself, the less crust you will eat.

This being said, if you strictly follow your ketogenic diet every day, it will be less of a problem for you to make a few exceptions when you are invited out. In the event that you aren't sure of the intended menu, such as when going to a friend's house for a meal, you can eat something at home before you leave. Doing so will allow you to limit your portions if you find that it is something you should not have.

Chapter 6:

Example Recipes

This section will give you some sample recipes with the serving size, number of calories and all the macronutrient gram counts for each serving.

Detoxing Liver Cleanse Smoothie

Due to the amount of carbohydrates in each serving of this smoothie, it is probably not a good idea to use it once you are in ketosis. However, this would be a good thing to add to your Pre-Keto diet a few days before you do begin following the ketogenic lifestyle. It will give you a jump start and get your liver used to breaking down more molecules and ease the transition of having to digest a greater amount of fats.

Ingredients

- 3 beets, shredded

- 3 carrots, shredded

- 2 c fresh spinach

- 1 c dandelion greens

- Zest of 1 lemon

- 1 lemon, peeled after zesting

- 1 apple, cored and sliced, leave the skin on

- 1 c red cabbage

- 2 tbsp coconut oil

- Enough filtered water to make it smooth

Directions

1. Add all beets and carrots to a high speed blender and pulse until the hard vegetables are broken down with enough water to keep it loose enough to move.

2. Add apple slices and cabbage with a bit more water. Pulse until just thin enough to move.

3. Add the remainder of the ingredients, pulse to break down.

4. Add enough water to fill blender canister to ¾ full.

5. Blend on high until liquified. More water can be added to reach the desired consistency.

6. Drink 8 ounces once or twice a day to boost your liver function and detox that vital organ.

7. **This blend will remain good for 2 days in the refrigerator. Store in a tightly closed, plastic container.**

Keto Bread

You can use these as a bun for your hamburgers or sausages. You can sprinkle them with a variety of seeds or herbs to add more flavor or crunch to them depending on what you are wanting them for. Adding a little artificial sweetener and cinnamon make them perfect for a quick breakfast or mid-morning snack topped with cream cheese too.

Ingredients

- 3 eggs

- 3.5 oz cream cheese

- pinch of salt

- ½ tbsp psyllium seed husks (opt)

- ½ tsp baking powder (opt)

Directions

1. Separate your eggs with the whites in one bowl and yolks in another.

2. Beat egg whites with salt, and artificial sweetener if making a sweet variety, into very stiff peaks.

3. Combine yolks and cream cheese well. Add the psyllium seed husk and baking powder at this time to make them more bread-like.

4. Gently fold the egg whites into the egg yolks. Make sure you keep the air in the egg whites.

5. Dip out 6 to 8 portions on a baking tray and spread out a little so that they rise uniformly.

6. Bake in the middle of your oven at 300 degrees for about 25 minutes or until golden brown.

Serving Size: 1 pieceCalories: 90Fats: 8gNet Carbs: 1gProtein: 4g

Keto Brown Butter Sauce

This sauce is perfect for pouring over meats and vegetables to give a little extra flavor or moisture should your recipe need such a thing. Try it on pork, fish or chicken or use it in place of gravy on mashed cauliflower.

Ingredients

- 4 tbsp butter

- 1 clove garlic

- ¼ c chicken broth

- 1/3 c cream

- ½ tsp salt

- ½ tsp pepper

Directions

1. Brown the butter in a pan by stirring it gently over medium heat.

2. Add garlic and cook for an additional minute to infuse the flavor.

3. Stir in chicken broth, cream, salt and pepper.

4. Lower heat to simmer. Stir occasionally 5-10 minutes until sauce has thickened.

5. Serve immediately.

6. Makes about ¾ cup of sauce.

Serving Size: 2 tbsp   Calories: 81   Fats: 8.8g   Net Carbs: 0.8g Protein: 0.4g

Keto-Friendly Pizza Crust

This is one of the absolute best low carb pizza crusts out there today. Whether you like a crispy or chewy crust, this one will be exactly what you're looking for. It tastes so much like the real thing that it will fool even the staunchest of wheat proponents in your life!

Ingredients

- 1 ½ c mozzarella and Cheddar cheeses, combined or just mozzarella alone

- 2 tbsp cream cheese

- 2 tbsp Parmesan cheese, freshly grated

- ¾ c almond flour

- 1 egg

- 1 tbsp Italian seasoning

- ½ tsp salt

Directions

1. Preheat your broiler.

2. In a microwave safe bowl, place mozzarella and cheddar cheeses. Heat until melted but not browned, about 30 seconds in the microwave.

3. When cheese is cool enough to handle, add remaining ingredients and knead together to form a soft, sticky dough. Use a little extra almond flour to help you form a ball if necessary.

4. Using a silpat or well greased parchment paper to line your baking sheet. Gently press into about a 12 inch round with your fingers. Wet your fingers if the cheese dough sticks to your hands. Make sure there are no holes.

5. Broil in oven for 5 minutes or until top is uniformly browned. Remove from beneath broiler. Use another pan to flip the crust over so that the browned top is now the bottom of the crust.

6. Broil an additional 5 minutes until the new side is uniformly browned.

7. Top with sauce and toppings, broil for 5 minutes or until cheese is bubbly and beginning to brown.

8. Allow to cool for 5-10 minutes before cutting.

9. Makes 4 servings, ¼ of the pizza.

Serving Size: ¼ pizza Calories: 290 Fats: 23.5g Net Carbs: 2.2g Protein: 18g

Amazing Keto Bread

Light and fluffy with enough of a bite to make you think you're cheating horribly on your diet. You'll think you're eating real wheat bread! Make a loaf or shape into buns to use for sandwiches. This recipe will remind you just why you switched to the ketogenic lifestyle.

Ingredients

- 1 ½ c almond flour or meal

- 1/3 c psyllium husk powder

- ½ c coconut flour

- ½ c flaxmeal
- 2 tsp garlic powder
- 2 tsp onion powder
- 2 tsp cream of tartar
- 1 tsp baking soda
- 1 tsp salt
- 2 tbsp erythritol (opt)
- 5 tbsp sesame, sunflower, flax or poppy seeds OR 1-2 tbsp caraway seeds
- 6 large egg whites
- 2 large eggs
- 2 c boiling water

Directions

1. Preheat your oven to 350 degrees.

2. In a large bowl, combine almond flour/meal, coconut flour, flaxmeal, psyllium, garlic and onion powders, erythritol, baking soda, cream of tartar and salt.

3. Add egg whites and eggs. Using a mixer, combine until dough is thick.

4. Add boiling water and mix well until combined.

5. Form a loaf and place into non-stick or greased loaf pan OR divide dough into 6 pieces to make sandwich buns. Place buns on non-stick or parchment lined baking sheet. Top loaf or buns with your choice of seeds, pressing seeds lightly into dough so they will stick.

6. Bake loaf for 75 minutes. Bake buns for 45-50 minutes.

7. Remove from oven and allow tray to cool before transferring loaf or buns to a cooling rack to cool to room temperature. If you will be using either loaf or buns within 2 days then they may be stored in an air proof container at room temperature. Otherwise, freeze for later use.

8. **Makes 1 loaf or 6 buns.**

**Notes about this recipe:

a) Do not use a silicon loaf pan when making this recipe as a loaf.

b) If you cannot find psyllium husk powder, use a coffee grinder or blender to process into a powder.

c) Do not waste the extra egg yolks from this recipe. Use them to make mayonnaise, Hollandaise sauce or lemon curd.

d) If your buns do not seem to rise, omit the whole eggs and use 8 egg whites only.

e) If the resulting buns are too moist, do not reduce the amount of water in the recipe because the psyllium will clump. Instead, place them in the oven at about 200 degrees for 30 minutes or so to allow them to dry out more. If the loaf is too moist, toast slices in your toaster.

f) Do not allow the dough to sit too long before cooking. It is best to put in the oven as soon as buns or loaf are formed.

g) If your buns or loaf take on a purple hue, this is due to the pre-made psyllium husk powder. It may not look appetizing but they are perfectly good.

h) **Be careful about not drinking enough when eating these buns.** The amount of psyllium husk powder can contribute to constipation in some people.

Serving Size: 2 slices/1 bun Calories: 242 Fats: 13.2g Net Carbs: 12.5g Protein: 12.1g

Bacon-Ceddar Omelet w/ Chives

This is a breakfast that anyone would enjoy, not just those on keto but the best thing is that it's the perfect start to your day and it doesn't take all that long to cook.

Ingredients

- 2 slices bacon, cooked

- 1 tsp bacon fat

- 2 large eggs, beaten

- 2 tbsp Cheddar cheese

- 1 tsp chives

- salt and pepper to taste

Directions

1. Cook your bacon, either in slices or cut it up and fry it in pieces.

2. Shred your cheese. You can use the pre-packaged shredded cheese but you must include the carbs that is added to prevent clumping in the package.

3. Mince your chives.

4. Heat bacon fat over low-medium heat.

5. Add beaten eggs when the fat sizzles. Season with salt, pepper and about half the chives.

6. When the edges have set, add your bacon and allow to cook for another 30 seconds.

7. Add most of the cheese to the center of your omelet. Flip one side up and hold in place to allow melting cheese to 'glue' it together. Repeat with other three sides to create a burrito-like form.

8. Turn off heat. Flip your omelet and allow to sit for 30 seconds or so to let the cheese melt.

9. Plate, garnish with leftover bacon bits, cheese and chives. Enjoy!

Serving Size: 1 omelet   Calories: 463   Fats: 39gNet Carbs: 1g
Protein: 24g

Triple Cheese, Bacon & Tomato Frittata

This recipe is so easy to make and with the right fillings, very satisfying. You can make it ahead of time and store it in the fridge to have it for a quick meal when you find yourself running short on time. This frittata will remain good for up to a week in the refrigerator.

Ingredients

- 1 c cherry tomatoes

- 6 slices bacon

- 10 eggs

- ¼ c heavy cream

- ½ c sharp cheddar cheese, shredded

- ¼ c Parmesan cheese

- ¼ c Feta cheese, crumbled

Directions

1. Cut bacon into bite sized pieces and fry in an oven-safe pan over medium heat until crispy. Cast iron is best since it can easily go from stovetop to oven without a problem. However, if you do not have a cast iron pan you may need to transfer all ingredients to a glass baking dish. Do not drain bacon.

2. Slice cherry tomatoes in half or quarters depending on size. Add to pan with crispy bacon and cook for 3-4 minutes.

3. In a large bowl, whisk eggs well. Add cream and combine thoroughly.

4. Add all cheeses to the egg mixture and mix well.

5. Pour egg and cheese mixture to the pan and allow to cook for about 2 minutes. Transfer the pan to the oven at 375 degrees for 20-25 minutes or until eggs are done in the center and top is lightly browned.

6. If you must transfer your ingredients to a glass baking dish, add the bacon and tomato mixture before pouring the eggs into the dish. You may need to cook for an additional 5 minutes or so to ensure doneness.

7. Makes 8 servings.

Serving Size: 1 piece   Calories: 210   Fats: 16.3g   Net Carbs: 2.8g Protein: 13.8g

Roasted Spaghetti Squash

This dish is a great low carbohydrate alternative to pasta. Spaghetti squash is full of nutrients like Vitamins A, B and C along with minerals, such as
calcium, magnesium, manganese and potassium. You don't need any special equipment to make the pasta strings since you can easily scrape it into 'noodles' with just a fork after it's been thoroughly cooked.

Ingredients

- 1 medium sized spaghetti squash

- 1 ½ tbsp butter

- 1 tbsp lemon juice

- ½ tsp dry basil

- ¼ c Parmesan cheese, shredded

- salt and pepper to taste

Directions

1. Cut your spaghetti squash in half length-wise and scoop out the seeds with a spoon.

2. Melt the butter and brush the insides of the squash including the cut section. Reserve any remaining butter for later use.

3. Sprinkle with salt and pepper.

4. Turn upside down on a baking sheet lined with parchment paper.

5. Roast at 375 degrees for 40 to 50 minutes, or until tender. Test tenderness with a fork.

6. When tender, shred the flesh into 'noodles' with a fork.

7. Combine remaining melted butter, lemon juice and basil. Pour over loosened 'noodles' and mix gently.

8. Top with Parmesan cheese and serve immediately.

9. Makes 3-4 servings.

Serving Size: 1 c Calories: 121 Fats: 8.7g Net Carbs: 7.6g Protein: 5.2g

Avocado-Tuna Melt Bites

If you've gone keto and find yourself missing a good tuna melt, now you don't have to miss that taste ever again! The crispy outside and the soft, creamy inside make you feel as though you've gotten your favorite non-keto sandwich back. Pair it with a keto-friendly salad and you have an easy way of getting your macros and eliminating any lingering hunger as you satisfy that desire for something that could easily knock you out of ketosis.

Ingredients

- 1 can (10oz) tuna, drained

- ¼ c mayonnaise

- 1 medium avocado, cubed

- ¼ c Parmesan cheese

- 1/3 c almond flour

- ½ tsp garlic powder

- ¼ tsp onion powder

- salt and pepper to taste

  ½ c coconut oil, for frying (some will be absorbed during frying to add to your fat intake)

-

Directions

1. Drain tuna and put in a bowl large enough to mix everything.

2. Combine tuna with mayonnaise, Parmesan cheese and spices together.

3. Slice your avocado in half, remove the pit and cut into cubes. Gently turn avocado pieces out into the tuna mixture and fold together without mashing the avocado too much.

4. Form the tuna mixture into balls and roll in almond flour until completely covered. Set aside to rest.

5. Heat coconut oil in a pan over medium heat.

6. Re-roll tuna balls in almond flour if they are tacky. Fry until crisp on all sides.

7. Remove from pan and serve immediately.

8. Makes about 12 balls.

Serving Size: 3 balls   Calories: 352   Fats: 36g   Net Carbs: 5.5g
Protein: 25g

Cheddar Stuffed, Bacon Wrapped Hot Dogs

This is a quick and easy lunch recipe that even your kids will love! It takes about 10 minutes to get this ready to go in the oven and tastes just the way you'd expect it to taste. Rich and savory!

Ingredients

- 2 hot dogs

- 12 slices bacon

- 2 oz Cheddar cheese

- ½ tsp garlic powder

- ½ tsp onion powder

- pepper to taste

Directions

1. Preheat your oven to 400 degrees.

2. Make a slit in each hot dog, do not cut into the ends.

3. Slice your Cheddar cheese into long, small rectangles. Stuff into the slits in the hot dogs.

4. Starting at one end, tightly wrap bacon around the hot dog. You will use 2 slices of bacon for each hot dog. Use toothpicks to keep the bacon from unrolling.

5. Set on a wire rack over a cookie sheet. Season with garlic powder, onion powder and pepper.

6. Bake for 35-40 minutes until bacon is crisped. You can also broil it for the last few minutes to crisp up the bacon.

7. Serve up with some delicious creamed spinach and watch your kids devour it.

Serving Size: 1 hot dog Calories: 380 Fats: 34.5g Net Carbs: 0.3g Protein: 16.8g

Chicken Pot Pie

This recipe is perfect for those cold winter days when you need something both filling and comforting to help you stay warm. Please be aware that this is a very high protein recipe so you will need to adjust your protein intake from other meals so that you don't end up falling out of ketosis due to excess protein turning into glucose.

Ingredients

- The Filling

- 6 chicken thighs, skinned and deboned
- 5 slices bacon
- 1 tsp onion powder
- 1 tsp garlic powder
- ¾ tsp celery seed
- 8 oz cream cheese
- 4 oz Cheddar cheese
- 6 c spinach
- ¼ c chicken broth
- salt and pepper to taste

-
  - 1/3 c almond flour
  - 3 tbsp psyllium husk powder
  - 3 tbsp butter
  - 1 egg
  - 2 oz cream cheese
  - 2 oz Cheddar cheese
  - ½ tsp paprika
  - ¼ tsp garlic powder
  - ¼ tsp onion powder
  - salt and pepper to taste

Directions

1. Cube chicken thighs. Season with salt and pepper.

2. Cut bacon into bite-sized pieces and add to a hot, oven-safe skillet. When bacon begins to render some fat add chicken pieces and spices. Continue

cooking until chicken and bacon are nicely browned.

3. Deglaze the pan with chicken broth. Add cream cheese and cheddar cheese. Stir well until cheese is melted.

4. Add spinach and allow to wilt.

5. While spinach is wilting, prepare crust as follows.

6. Combine all dry ingredients in one bowl and both cheeses in a separate bowl.

7. Microwave cheese about 30 seconds or until melted.

8. Add egg and melted cheese mixture to the dry ingredients and mix well.

9. Using a silpat, form the crust into a circle about the same size as the pan.

10.   When the spinach has wilted, mix everything together. Invert the silpat over the pan and gently place crust over ingredients in the pan. Don't worry about the crust tearing as you can fix that with your fingers.

11. Place in oven and cook for 15 minutes at 375 degrees. Serve immediately.

12.   Makes 8 servings.

Serving Size: 1 slice   Calories: 505   Fats: 34.1g   Net Carbs: 2.8g
Protein: 42.6

Slow Cooker Braised Beef Roast

The best thing about bone-in meat is that you're stewing the meat
into tenderness but also a large amount of bone and marrow which
will add to the nutrition and flavor of this dish. This recipe is best
when you use oxtail but that is not always readily available so use a
fatty, bone in chuck roast to get a similar flavor. This recipe makes
3 servings and requires guar gum as a thickening agent. If you
have 7g of carbs available, you can substitute corn starch for the
guar gum.

Ingredients

- 2-3 lbs bone-in oxtails or chuck roast

- 2 c beef broth

- 1/3 c butter

- 2 tbsp soy sauce

- 1 tbsp fish sauce

- 3 tbsp tomato paste

- 1 tsp onion powder

- 1 tsp fresh garlic, minced

- ½ tsp ground ginger

- 1 tsp thyme

- salt and pepper to taste

- ½ tsp guar gum

Directions

1. Place your oxtails or roast in your slow cooker.

2. In a saucepan on the stove top, combine beef broth, soy sauce, fish sauce, tomato paste and butter. Heat until butter is melted and all ingredients are combined.

3. Season your oxtail or roast with onion powder, garlic, ginger, thyme, salt and pepper.

4. Pour hot liquids over the meat in the slow cooker.

5. Cook on low for 6-7 hours.

6. Once cooked, remove meat and set aside. Separate meat from bones.

7. Using an immersion blender, add guar gum to the leftover juices in the slow cooker. Blend until a slightly thickened gravy forms.

8. Serve with Mashed Cheddar Cauliflower Mock-Potatoes.

Serving Size: 1/3 of the meat Calories: 433 Fats: 29.7g Net Carbs: 3.2g Protein: 28.3g

Mashed Cheddar Cauliflower Mock-Potatoes

This dish is perfect for anyone following a ketogenic diet when they have that potato craving. Creamy and savory, you'd never know it wasn't Cheddar mashed potatoes.

Ingredients

- 1 head cauliflower, trimmed and cleaned

- 2 cloves garlic, peeled

- 1 bay leaf

- ½ c Cheddar cheese, shredded

- 2 tbsp butter

- 2 tbsp sour cream

- salt and pepper to taste

Directions

1. Using a steamer or pot with a steaming basket, place cauliflower in basket and garlic and bay leaf in the water. Steam cauliflower until tender.

2. Remove cauliflower and place in a blender. Retrieve garlic cloves and transfer to blender. Discard bay leaf.

3. Add Cheddar cheese, butter and sour cream to blender.

4. Blend mixture to desired consistency.

5. Season with salt and pepper. Serve immediately.

6. Makes 4 servings.

Serving Size: ½ cup   Calories: 139   Fats: 11.8g   Net Carbs: 2.7g Protein: 5.2g

Stuffed Pork Tenderloin

Whether you're going low-carb or not, this particular recipe will just hit the spot. The herbs and spices come through with each bite and the sausage-mushroom-spinach stuffing makes you not miss the traditional bread stuffing.

Ingredients

- Pork Loin

  - 2 lb pork tenderloin

  - 3 tsp salt

  - 1 tsp pepper

  - 1 ½ tsp onion powder

  - 1 tsp garlic powder

  - 2 tsp thyme

  - 2 tsp rosemary

-

  - 1 lb ground pork sausage

  - 6 oz baby portabella mushrooms

- 3 oz spinach

- ½ tsp thyme

- ½ tsp rosemary

- ¼ tsp garlic powder

- ¼ tsp onion powder

- salt and pepper to taste

Directions

1. Butterfly the pork tenderloin.

a)   Hold the knife blade flat so that it is parallel to the cutting board. Make a lengthwise cut into the center of the tenderloin. Don't cut all the way through the opposite edge so that the flaps remain attached.

b)   Open the tenderloin as you would a book.

c)   Cover the meat with plastic wrap. Using a meat mallet, rolling pin or heavy flat-bottomed pan, pound the meat to the desired thickness.

2. Season both sides of the flattened pork loin with salt, pepper, onion powder, garlic powder, thyme and rosemary.

3. Slice the mushrooms.

4. Preheat your oven to 400 degrees.

5. In a large skillet, crumble the sausage and fry over medium heat. Make sure to break it up as it browns.

6. Add mushrooms, salt, pepper, onion powder, garlic powder, thyme, and rosemary when the sausage is cooked through. Stir to

   combine.

7. Add the spinach to the pan and allow to wilt. Mix well so that all ingredients are distributed evenly.

8. Pour sausage mixture over the top of the tenderloin and spread it out evenly.

9. Roll the pork loin up and wrap in butchers netting or tie with butchers string. Place in roasting pan, seam side down.

   10. Cook at 400 degrees for 50-60 minutes or until meat thermometer reaches 140 degrees internal temperature.

11. When pork loin is cooked through, remove from oven and allow to rest for 10-15 minutes. Slice and serve with your favorite sides.

12. Makes 6 servings.

Serving Size: 1/6 of the meat Calories: 439 Fats: 21.6g Net Carbs: 4.3g Protein: 52.5g

Banana-Chia Seed Pudding

You might not think that chia seeds would be so filling, but they are extremely nutritious and almost completely fiber. This pudding takes about 5 minutes to prepare. You just let it sit in the refrigerator overnight to thicken and breakfast will be ready straight out of the fridge.

Ingredients

- 1 can coconut milk, full fat

- 1 medium sized banana, ripe to over ripe (the browner the better)

- ½ tsp cinnamon

- ½ tsp salt

- 1 tsp vanilla extract

- ¼ c Chia seeds

Directions

1. In a medium sized bowl, mash your banana until soft enough to stir. The darker brown it is, the more oil will come out. This is used as the sweetener for your pudding and is surprisingly low in carbohydrates for a fruit.

2. Add the remaining ingredients and stir until combined.

3. Cover tightly and store in the refrigerator overnight.

4. Makes 2-3 servings.

Serving Size: ½ cup   Calories: 327   Fats: 32.9g   Net Carbs: 4.8g Protein: 3.6g

Lemon Cheesecake Pudding

This recipe is for those days when you need something just sweet enough but is still satisfying.

Ingredients

- 8 oz cream cheese, softened

- ½ c heavy cream

- 4-5 packets artificial sweetener, Stevia or erythritol

- ½ tsp lemon extract

Directions

1. Combine all ingredients well with a hand mixer.

2. Spoon into pudding dishes.

3. Makes 4 servings.

Serving Size: 1/3 cup   Calories: 251   Fats: 25.3g   Net Carbs: 4g
Protein: 4.6g

Double Peanut Butter Balls

There's just something about peanut butter that is absolutely addicting. These dessert balls are perfectly fine without additional sweetening but you can decide if you want to add it or leave it out. You can give it a little twist with the nuts that you garnish this dessert with as well, roast them before using or dust them with different spices; cinnamon, vanilla, nutmeg or cardamom. It's best if you use homemade nut butters but so long as you keep track of the carbs added to the commercially made nut butters, you can get away with using those instead.

Ingredients

- 2 tbsp homemade peanut butter

- 2 tbsp homemade almond butter

- 2 tbsp butter, do not melt

- 2 tbsp heavy cream

- 1 ½ tsp granulated sweetening

- 4 drops liquid sweetening

Directions

1. In a small bowl, combine all ingredients.

2. Using a fork to incorporate all ingredients, be sure not to break down the butter completely. Small bits of butter in this mixture will give you little changes in taste and texture as you enjoy it.

3. Set aside in the freezer for 20-40 minutes. You want it to hold up to handling when you roll it out.

4. Portion into quarters. Roll each quarter into a ball.

5. Garnish with chiffenade mint and chopped peanuts.

Serving Size: 1 ball   Calories: 177   Fats: 16.8g   Net Carbs: 1.8g   Protein: 4.4g

Each of the recipes found here give you an idea of what you can enjoy on the ketogenic diet. You don't even need to give up your sweets! You just have to find a different way to make them and the internet is full of such recipes. Bon Apetit!

Conclusion

So now we reach the end of this book and you've learned a lot about the ketogenic diet and how you can make it work for you. Welcome to the world of better health!

The testing that has been done on the ketogenic diet has shown that it is safe and that it actually works better than nearly all traditional diet plans. Whether you are simply wanting to lose weight or you are making this transition to improve a chronic disease that will respond to metabolic changes, the ketogenic lifestyle will make it so much easier.

It is hoped that you will find the information contained within these pages helpful and intriguing enough to make you want to learn more about this particular diet plan. The internet is full of informative websites that will give you more scientific information as well as thousands of books and e-books available for purchase. However, if you do choose to read websites or e-books on this subject please be certain to do your research. The worst thing that could happen with your health on this diet is to get information from a less than credible source.

This doesn't mean that you shouldn't follow the recipes posted on someone's blog, just that you should be sure that they have been following this diet for a while before trusting that they have fully vetted their information and recipes. That is the hardest thing to do, vetting recipes so that you don't end up sabotaging yourself by getting too many carbohydrates or too little protein.

And, finally, stick to the plan! Ketosis is something that happens to your body and it is a wonderful thing. Unfortunately, you just can't afford to cheat on a regular basis. As mentioned earlier, you shouldn't beat yourself up if you aren't quite as careful about counting those macros but that doesn't mean that you can have that delicious baked potato or deep dish, Chicago style pizza your friends ordered. With some will power and the fact that you are feeling better, you will find that making the keto choices are really quite easy.

Remember that the keto diet allows you to find things that satisfy you so feel free to change up the kinds of foods you eat. Research recipes containing foods you love. Experiment with making recipes you find here and on the internet or in cookbooks and see if you can make them better. The ketogenic diet isn't just about eating better – it's about eating *well*!

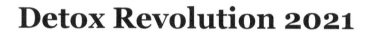

Detox Revolution 2021

Table of Contents

Introduction

Thank you for downloading my book. Because you downloaded it you are clearly looking for more information on detox cleanses and how they work, how they can help you to drop weight, smooth out those wrinkles and help you feel much more refreshed and healthy. But why do we need to detox? Doesn't the human body already do it for us naturally?

Well, yes it does to a certain degree but it can only be effective if your body isn't overloaded with toxins and pollutants and that's where the trouble lies these days. While technology and science have brought no end of improvements to our lives, they have also filled the air we breathe with pollutants and so many of us are finding that we are taking in more toxins than our bodies can possibly remove.

Toxins come from everywhere – in the air we breathe, the water we drink and the ground we walk on. They come from the many synthetic materials that we use or wear on a daily basis and they come from the food we eat. You could argue that you eat a healthy diet but you would be shocked to know just how many toxins are laced through the meat you eat, the seafood, even the vegetables. And, for those who eat a "junk" diet, well, your bodies really are overloaded.

Would it really surprise you to know that your food is laced with chemicals, pesticides, metals? Processed food is especially bad for this but it's also in the water you drink as well. There are more chronic illnesses in evidence now than there ever has been and because of the sheer number of different toxins passing into the body every day, it's become impossible for us to remove them naturally.

With this book, my aim is to show you why you need to detox and how to do it safely. I will tell you what builds up in the body, where it comes from and how to remove it with some very simple steps, steps that anyone can take. I will tell you what foods you should eat and what you shouldn't and I will also give you a couple of recipes to take away with you and try. So, without any further waiting, let's dive in and see what's what.

Chapter 1:

What is Detoxification?

Detox is short for detoxification and it is a natural process whereby the body removes toxins from our blood and our organs. Toxins are, to put it simply, poisons. Anything that can cause harm to the body tissues is a toxin, including waste products that come from cell activity – waste products like ammonia, homocysteine, and lactic acid. Add to that the man-made toxins we are exposed to on a daily basis and it's easy to see how our bodies can become overloaded.

In order to eliminate toxins from the body, the intestines, liver, kidneys, skin, blood, lungs, and our lymphatic systems all work together to turn harmful toxins into harmless compounds that can be eliminated out of the body, through sweat, urine and bowel elimination.

Because of the sheer number of toxins we are exposed to our bodies are struggling to remove them efficiently. If the body cannot use what we ingest nutritionally or eliminate it naturally, it will remain in our blood and lymphatic systems, eventually moving into body tissues, and staying put.

Detoxification is the process of cleansing the body of these toxins and giving your system a boost it so desperately needs.

What is a Toxin?

Toxins are any compounds that affect cell function or cell structure in an adverse manner and includes:

- Heavy Metals – Mercury, lead, aluminum – accumulate in the kidneys, brain and immune system

- Liver Toxicants – Alcohol, drugs, pesticides, toxic chemicals, food additives – constant exposure can cause severe liver damage

- Microbial Toxins – Toxins absorbed by yeast and bacteria that lives in the intestines – can cause serious disruptions to normal bodily functions

- Products of the Breakdown of Protein Metabolism – ammonia and urea – can overload the kidneys, especially if you eat too much protein

Every day we are exposed to herbicides, pesticides, food additives, solvents and so many other toxins and, most of the time, we don't even realize it. It's not like you know you are breathing in or ingesting these toxins because you can see or taste them – if you did, you wouldn't do it.

Asthma, chronic fatigue, lupus, fibromyalgia, migraines, and multiple sclerosis can all be attribute to constant exposure to these toxins. Studies have shown that people who suffer from any of these have experienced a reversal of their symptoms after they have been through a total cleansing detoxification process.

A full detox process will improve your health in so many ways by:

- Removing heavy metals – including mercury and lead

- Detoxifying – the liver, kidneys, blood and other body organs

- Recharging your immune system – through introducing powerful antioxidants into your body

- Replenishing friendly bacteria – especially the most important ones in the intestines

10 Signs That Your Liver Needs a Detox

You already know by now that your liver is one of the most powerful organs in your body and, next to the heart is one of the hardest working. Your liver has two jobs – detoxifying your body and working as a digestive organ. In today's modern world, most of us have a liver that is overworked and cannot cope. Unfortunately, most of us don't listen to the signs so the following 10 signs should help you to realize that your liver is crying out to you for relief:

- Bloating around the abdomen
- Pain around the liver area
- Too much belly or abdominal fat
- You struggle to digest fatty foods
- You have had your gallbladder out
- You suffer with acid reflux or heartburn
- You have liver spots on your skin
- You sweat excessively and overheat quickly
- You have acne, rosacea or dry blotchy and itchy skin
- You put on weight unexpectedly and can't lose it even on a calorie controlled diet There are a number of other signs that will give it away as well, including:
- High blood pressure
- Fatigue
- High triglycerides and cholesterol
- Depression
- Mood swings
- Sleep apnea
- Snoring

- Yellow fatty lumps around the eyes

These are all signs that your liver is struggling and that you need to detox, change your diet and shake up your lifestyle in order for your liver to heal. What these signs are telling you is that your liver is blocked up with unhealthy fat, if it's extreme, it's called fatty liver disease. The cells in your liver that are used as filters become swollen up with fat and cannot filter the rubbish out. Remember that the blood is filtered through the liver, cleaned out and sent back to the heart. If you don't clean your liver out, you are sending toxic blood back up to your heart that can cause damage to the cardiovascular system, the immune system and it can cause rapid aging.

How Does Fatty Liver Happen?

There are two ways – the first is through alcohol and the second is through diet. People who don't drink can get NAFD – Non Alcoholic Fatty Liver Disease and this is generally attributed to following a diet that is high in carbohydrates and processed or sugary foods.

What Else?

As we already talked about earlier, there are such high levels of toxins all around these days that we can't escape them. They are on our food in the form of pesticides, in our water, in food preservatives, electromagnetic radiation and heavy metals. They come into our blood through the food, the air, even through home cleaning and personal care products. They move in to the bowel, the kidneys, the liver, fat tissue and the lymphatic system and they build up, stopping our bodies from taking in the nutrients, proteins, carbohydrates and using them effectively. It even reduces that amount of oxygen in your blood and puts you into a state of low energy, susceptible to disease.

Because the liver is working so hard to try to filter these toxins out, it can't do all its others jobs, resulting in a weight gain and a struggle to lose it again.

REMEMBER

Your skin is the single biggest organ in your body and what goes on it goes through it. The simple rule of thumb is this – if you wouldn't eat it, don't put it on your skin. Even those products that are labeled as organic might have used toxins in the preserving process so try to go for those with essential preservatives.

If you can make your own skin products using coconut oil, organic shea butter, olive oil, jojoba oil and essential oils.

Be aware that lots of things we take for granted these days emit electromagnetic fields, such as cordless phones, mobile phones, Wi-Fi, airplanes and x-rays. When you are sleeping, keep all electronic things at least 8 feet away from you, if not in another room.

The next thing you must do is look at your diet and eliminate the foods that are harming your liver. Get rid of processed foods, those that are high in sugars and simple carbohydrates. Eat more raw food, such as vegetables and fruits and, if you do cook, don't overcook foods. Get rid of your microwave, as this does nothing but destroy anything good that was in the food.

Make the switch to high quality oils, such as olive or coconut and eliminate the lower quality oils.

Don't eat animal products that are not grass-fed or free range.

If you have at least three of the symptoms listed above, cut alcohol out of your diet altogether.

Add supportive foods to your diet – lots of brightly colored fruits and vegetables and dark leafy greens. At least 30- 40% of your diet should be raw vegetables and fruits. These are useful because they have living enzymes in them, as well as vitamin C, phyto-nutrients and natural antibiotics. If you don't like eating them raw, juice them or add them to a smoothie.

You should also try to eat foods that are naturally fermented, such as sauerkraut, apple cider vinegar, cultured vegetables and yogurt. The other important nutrients that your body needs are:

- **Vitamin K** – from dark leafy vegetables

- **Arginine** – legumes, oats, carob, walnuts, seeds and wheat germ. These help the liver to detoxify ammonia

- **Antioxidants** – raw carrot, beetroot, celery, apple, pear, dandelion juices and green drinks that are made contain spirulina and chlorella. Also found in fresh kiwi and citrus fruits

- **Selenium** – Brazil nuts, brown rice, kelp, seafood, molasses, garlic, whole grains, onion, wheat germ

- **Methionine** – Legumes, fish, eggs, onion, garlic, seeds, meat

- **Essential fatty acids** – cod liver oil seafood, fish oil. Seafood can be frozen, fresh or canned and includes salmon, sardines, mackerel, trout, tuna, blue mussels, mullet, herring, calamari and blue eye cod. Avocado, raw nuts, seeds, whole grains, legumes, green vegetables, such as spinach, kale, beet greens. Eggplant, cold pressed seed and vegetable oils, fresh ground seeds, evening primrose oil, starflower oil and blackcurrant seed oil. EFAs are needed to keep the cells in the body healthy and you need to consume them in plentiful amounts to keep your liver functioning properly. This is why low fat diets are generally not good for weight control, health and liver function.

- **Natural sulfur** – eggs, onions, garlic, leeks, shallots, broccoli, cabbage, cauliflower, Brussels sprouts

Finally, in order to help your liver get back to tip top condition you should use supportive nutrients and herbs. The B complex vitamins are important for liver function, as are natural beta-carotenes, and vitamins C and E. Globe artichokes; milk thistle, dandelion and turmeric are also good for helping the liver.

What is a Detox Cleanse?

Most of us assume that detox is primarily a treatment for dependence on drugs or alcohol. However, a detox cleanse is also used as a method of losing weight, clearing the skin and generally improving health. A detox cleanse is a short-term way of rebooting your life, of removing all those chemicals and toxins from your body and giving you a clean slate to start over with.

Detox diets are not long-term solutions. If you were to follow a detox diet for any longer than a few days your body would be deprived of essential nutrients and you would not be getting balance of the food groups that you need for optimum health.

You can follow a detox diet for up to one week but you must then move on to a healthy diet. There is no harm in repeating the detox on a regular basis – some people kick start their bodies with a one week cleanse and then do a three day cleanse once a month afterwards – this will not harm you provided you are eating a sensible diet in between times.

A detox cleanse will:

- Drastically reduce the amount of chemicals that you ingest

- Place more importance on the foods that contain the nutrients, vitamins and essential antioxidants that your body needs to detoxify itself naturally

- Contain food groups that are high in water content and fiber, both of which help to draw out and eliminate the toxins – this works because by eating more fiber and drinking more water, the frequency of urination and bowel movements you experience will increase.

- Help to prevent chronic diseases. Toxins that we encounter in the environment are responsible for so many neurological diseases, cancers, strokes, heart disease, and so many more. While our bodies do naturally detox, they can't cope when they are overloaded so a detox gives us a boost and helping hand.

• Enhances your immune system function. If your immune system has been compromised, you are significantly more likely to catch flu, colds and other viruses, which affect your productivity and your quality of life. Detoxing on a regular basis helps build up strength in the immune system and helps to fight off infection.

• Drop those pounds. A healthy body has a natural ability to burn off excess fat but an overload of toxins stops that from working. As we all know, a number of chronic diseases are linked with weight gain, including heart disease, diabetes and high blood pressure. Detoxing removes the toxins in the fat cells and increases your metabolism rate.

• Slows down premature aging. Heavy metals and free radicals are partly responsible for rapid aging and detox will eliminate those from the body. This means your body will increase more nutrients, including vitamins and antioxidants that help to fight off oxidative stress.

• Improve your quality of life. Put simply, if our bodies are overloaded with toxins, they will not function as they should. You may experience pain in your joints, a lack of energy, trouble sleeping, headaches and problems digesting your food. Detoxing can improve your memory function and ease depression as well.

• Increase your energy. A detox will give you more physical, mental and emotional energy and you will sleep much better.

• Improve your skin quality. Toxins cause acne, weak hair and weak nails as well as making us look pale and ill. Regular detox cleansing will improve all of that and give you back a healthy glow.

●   Improve your emotional and mental clarity. This will allow you to deal with more, make better decisions and think much clearer. You will also see things differently and won't be prone to seeing a small problem as something that is insurmountable.

●   Restore the balance to your body. Overloads of toxins and bad foods stop your hormonal, digestive and nervous systems from working together in harmony and make you ill. Detoxing restores the balance.

Chapter 2:

Who Shouldn't Try a Detox Cleanse?

While detox cleanses are generally safe, you should consult your doctor first. People who definitely should not undertake a detox cleanse are pregnant or nursing women, young children, or anyone who has a disease of the kidneys or liver. This is also not intended to be used as a way of treating alcohol or drug related dependencies – these must be treated in the correct manner.

If you suffer with a persistent cough, pain in the muscles, indigestion, or insomnia, do not assume that it's because your body is overloaded with toxins. It may well be but you do need to see a doctor first to ensure that there is nothing more serious going on.

Side Effects of a Detox Cleanse

The single most common side effect of a detox cleanse is a headache and this can last for a couple of days. This is mainly down to a withdrawal from caffeine. To avoid this, before you start a detox cleanse, gradually decrease how much caffeine you drink so it isn't such a shock to the system.

Other side effects can cause bad diarrhea, which will lead to a loss of electrolytes and dehydration. If you eat too much fiber, the opposite can occur – chronic constipation. To avoid this you must drink plenty of fluids. You may experience tiredness, hunger, irritability and an outbreak of acne but these are extreme cases.

For these reasons, you should try to start your detox cleanse on a weekend or take some time off work. It's only for a few days and you will feel so much better afterwards as your body clears the rubbish out and makes way for good health.

How to Deal With the Symptoms of a Detox

Not everyone will feel great to start with on a detox and, if you find that you need a bit of a push to get past a sticking point, these tips will help you:

- **Drink**. I already said above to make sure you are drinking enough water to maintain your hydration levels. This also helps to stop you becoming constipated. A detox can involve a high level of fiber, which can stop you from going so get drinking!

- **Sweat** – Toxins in our bodies are removed in three ways – through the digestive tract, through the lungs and through the skin. Work up a sweat through doing some light exercise and the toxins will exit your body through your pores. As well as that, your lymph fluid will get moving again. You could also use a wet or dry sauna or a steam room to produce the same results.

- **Have a Massage** – massages are good for sore muscles but they also stimulate the lymph fluid and get it flowing again. Your lymphatic system is vital to get rid of waste that the body doesn't need. Blood and lymph fluid circulation can help you to recover from the symptoms of detox a lot quicker. You can also add Epsom salts to your bath and soak in it for half an hour after dry brushing dead skin cells off.

- **Find a Substitute** - cravings are tough to deal with but instead of heading for the chocolate, pick a piece of fruit or a handful of nuts, something from the list of foods that you are allowed to eat. If you really do crave chocolate, add some raw cacao to a smoothie. If you crave salt, add kelp seasoning to food.

If you are missing fat, eat an avocado or add it to your smoothie, with a spot of coconut oil. In time, you can train your brain to look for healthy alternatives to processed foods.

- **Rest** – A couple of days in to your detox cleanse, you may start feeling a little fatigued. Don't try to fight it, you will only feel worse. Respect your limits and listen to your body. If you are tires, rest, sneak a ten-minute power nap on your lunch break if you can. Give it a couple of days and you will have so much energy you won't know what to do with it.

- **Breathe** – You can help to release toxins by learning deep breathing and yoga exercises. Also, deep belly breathing will help to stimulate your lymph flow as well as calming your body and your mind

5 Reasons You Need a Detox Cleanse

When we talk about detox, many of us automatically envisage hunger, deprivation, weird and wonderful juices and drinks. We may wonder if it is worth all the effort and the suffering. You don't need to suffer with a detox cleanse – yes, you may get a headache and you may get a touch of diarrhea but only if you don't do it right, if you jump straight into it without preparing yourself first.

You might also be asking yourself if you really need a detox cleanse so, if you are one of those take a look at these 5 reasons why you do need one – I bet you can identify with at least one of them:

1. You have FLC Syndrome

FLC stands for, to put it bluntly, Feel Like Crap. When you wake up you don't feel awake. You have no energy; you drag yourself out of the bed and through your morning routine without any sense of joy or vitality. Think about this– do you suffer with fatigue, allergies, digestive problems, brain fog, headaches? If you do then barring any other medical issues, a detox can help you to get rid of that FLC syndrome.

2. You struggle to lose weight and/or keep it off

Yes, I know, everyone will tell you that losing weight and keeping it off is nothing more than decreasing your calories and increasing your exercise. OK, so that can help but it isn't the whole story. For instance, did you know that not all calories are equal? That the calories in flour and sugar are totally different to other calories? These calories trigger overeating and a type of addiction. They raise your insulin levels and increase inflammation in the body, that's why you store fat in your belly, and you never feel full up. A detox removes those calories from the equation and teaches you a completely new way of eating that helps you drop the pounds and keep them off while feeling full and eating less.

3. You get really bad cravings for sugar and carbs

Flour and sugar are addictive; there is no two ways about it. It's been proven time and time again. Yet, are we not quick to accuse an overweight person of being lazy? Add to this that most of the foods you eat containing sugar and flour are processed and you get an additional overload of chemicals and toxins that you really don't need. But it is these toxins that cause the cravings and a detox cleanse removes that instantly.

Just as an aside, it may interest you to know that sugar is more than 8 times more addictive than a drug like cocaine and using sheer willpower to lose weight simply will not work. You need to detox your body and train yourself to understand that you do not need sugar or any processed floury sugary foods whatsoever.

4. You have never done a detox in your entire life

Most of us haven't but we should. It's only a few days here and there, nothing in the grand scheme of things. Just a few days to fill your body with clean food and get rid of the buildup of toxins. If you think you feel healthy now, wait until you have been through a detox cleanse and then tell me what healthy feels like!

5. Your body needs a break

And so do you. The way we live our lives these days is not conducive to good health − we sleep too little, we eat too much junk, we don't exercise enough and we get stressed out. And we don't take enough time out for us. One of the best ways to reset your life is a detox cleanse. You are only a few days away from feeling the best you have ever felt, a few days away from being happy and healthy again.

Five Ways to Detox

If you want to lose weight, lose the wrinkles, and feel great again, you need to undergo a detox. Choose from these five ways to kick start your life again:

1. Go cold turkey

This is the only way to handle a true physiological addiction. If you are addicted to junk foods, the only way to get them out of your system completely is to stop it. Go on a 3, 5 or 7-day detox and reset the hormones and neurotransmitters in your body, Get rid of the toxins, eliminate cravings and increase your metabolism. I'm not just talking about food that you eat either. Think about what you drink. Did you know that the latte you grab on the way into work has more sugar in it than a can of soda? All that does is makes you want to eat.

Check your labels − cut out anything that has Trans fats, hydrogenated fats, and monosodium glutamate (MSG). In fact, don't eat anything that comes in a box, a packet, even a can and stick to eating whole fresh foods. The best way to detox quickly is to eliminate grains from your diet for a week and cut out sugar and alcohol.

2. Power up with protein

Protein is the best thing you can eat, at every single meal, most importantly at breakfast. Protein helps to balance out the cravings for sugar so start the day with eggs or a good protein smoothie. Eat seeds, nuts, fish, chicken or eggs at every meal. Make sure you use organic grass fed meats and butters.

3. Don't limit the good carbs

Vegetables contain carbs Fruit contains carbs although a lot of fruits are high in sugars as well. Avoid starchy carbs and fill up of greens – kale, spinach, beet greens, broccoli, cauliflower, and collards. Eat asparagus, mushrooms, zucchini, onions, green beans, tomatoes and fennel. Cut out potatoes, squash, beets – just for 1 week and see how it makes you feel. I guarantee you will lose weight, you will look younger and you will feel great and you will never want to go back to the way you used to eat.

4. Eat fat not sugar

For so many years we have been told that fat is bad for us but now, at long last, nutritionists and doctors have finally understood the difference between good fat and bad fat and just how important the first one is in our diets. Good fat fills you up and evens out the glucose in your blood. You don't get the insulin spikes or the sugar highs and lows. Eat oily fish, butter, nuts, seeds, olive oil, avocadoes, all excellent sources of omega 3 and 6 fats. And they are not called essential for nothing!

5. Forget willpower, use friend power instead

If you are looking to lose weight and feel great then forget willpower. It will not work. What will work is doing a detox cleanse with a friend. You have the right kind of support and the push you need to keep going and you can compare results!

Detox for Fast Weight Loss

Let's answer one of the most common questions asked – do detox diets really work? Do they live up to all that hype? The answer is yes, they do work, but only if you follow them correctly. Most detox diets are short – between 3 and 21 days and they are highly calorie restricted. They cut out the fast food, the processed food, the alcohol, sugar, caffeine and some of them will even eliminate wheat, dairy and meat. Most of them are heavily focused on vegetables and fruit, sometimes in their raw form and sometimes in a juice or a smoothie.

You can lose a significant amount of weight doing a detox but you must keep one thing in mind. Most of the initial weight loss will be water and if you go straight back to your old eating habits afterwards, the weight will pile back on. You should use a detox cleansing diet as the starting point of a new way of life, a new way of eating, although you can use one just to drop a dress size beer a big event if you want.

One thing that all detox diets contain is cleansing elements. They contain fluid and fiber, both of which help eliminate metabolic waste out of the body. Certain herbs and nutritional supplements may be included to help stimulate the enzymes in the liver that break the toxins down. When it comes down to the wire, we all know, deep down, that a whole food diet is better than a juice fast but you can start your regime with a juice diet and ease yourself in to a whole food diet. Whole foods help to improve your metabolism, support your liver and your colon and you can lose weight easily without having to starve yourself for days.

Detox diets are also very good for helping to identify the foods that are taking their energy, food allergies and to help cut the cravings for bad foods. The real benefit to any diet comes a couple of weeks after starting, which is when the fat loss really begins to start happening. A detox diet, followed by a whole food diet is going to have more effect than a 3-day detox followed by you going back to your normal eating habits.

What I am going to give you now is a way to drop a quick 5 lbs. to lighten the load a bit – without starving yourself! The following meal plan will fill you up with metabolism boosting carbs, helping you to burn off fat while you stay fuller for longer. Follow the plan for 5 days and drop 5 lbs. You can extend it to 7 days but no more.

Either eat these meals every day for 5 days or make up your own meal plan using similar ingredients; this is just to start you off.

Breakfast Banana Shake Ingredients:

- 1 large banana
- 12 oz. 1% milk – low fat
- 2 tsp honey
- ½ cup ice

Preparation

- Chop the banana
- Put the ice in the blender, followed by all other ingredients
- Blend until smooth

Lunch

Pecan Crusted Goats Cheese Salad, Pomegranate Vinaigrette Ingredients:

- 4 oz. polenta, cut into slices about ½ inch thick
- 1 oz. goats cheese
- 1 tbsp. pecans, chopped
- 2 tbsp. pomegranate juice
- 1 tsp olive oil
- 1 tsp Dijon mustard
- 3 cups fresh spinach
- ½ cup carrot, shredded

Preparation

- Heat up a nonstick pan over a medium heat. Spray cooking oil over the polenta and put them in the pan, cook for 5 minutes. Turn the slices and cook for a further 5 minutes

- Make a patty out of the goats cheese and coat it with the chopped pecans

- Mix the pomegranate juice, mustard and oil together in a small bowl; which to combine thoroughly

- Put the spinach and carrot onto a serving plate, top with the polenta and the cheese

- Sprinkle vinaigrette over and enjoy!

Dinner

Black Bean, Brown Rice, Avocado and Chicken Wrap
Ingredients

- ½ tsp salt

- ¼ tsp black pepper

- 1 1/3 cups black beans, low sodium, drained and properly rinsed

- 1 tsp chili powder

- ½ tsp cumin

- ¼ tsp chili flakes

- 8 oz. chicken breast, grilled and sliced

- 4 whole wheat wraps

- 1 1/3 cup brown rice, cooked

- 1 small shredded carrot

- ½ avocado, stone removed and diced

- 1 Roma tomato, seeds removed and chopped

- Hot sauce – optional

Preparation

- Mix the first 6 ingredients together and toss
- Put a wrap flat on a clean surface
- Spoon 1/3 cup of rice on the bottom of it and add 1/3 cup bean mix, 2 oz. chicken and ¼ cup carrot
- Add 1 tbsp. of avocado and 2 tbsp. tomato
- Seal the wrap up, cut in half and serve straight away; season with hot sauce if desired

Snack

Greek Yoghurt Parfait Ingredients

- 3 cups of fat free plain Greek yogurt
- 1 tsp vanilla extract
- 4 tsp honey
- 28 segments of clementine
- ¼ cup unsalted dry roasted shelled and chopped pistachios

Preparation

- Mix the yogurt and the honey together
- Spoon 1/3 cup of the mix into each of 4 parfait glasses
- Add ½ tsp honey to the top, with 5 sections of clementine and ½ tbsp. nuts
- Add another 1/3 cup of the honey and yogurt mixture on to the top of each
- Add a further ½ tsp of honey, 2 more segments of clementine and ½ tbsp. nuts
- Serve straight away

All-Day Drink

Fat Flushing Cooler Ingredients
- 8 cups of brewed green tea
- As many slices of lime, orange and lemon as you want

Preparation
- Pour the green tea into a pitcher
- Add the fruit slices
- Drink it warm or refrigerate and serve over ice
- You can drink a pitcher of this every day

Detox for Anti-Aging

To detox your skin to prevent rapid aging, you do not have to spend a small fortune on creams or plastic surgery. The best way to detox your skin and give you back that youthful complexion and glow is to eat the right foods. You need foods that are full of antioxidant nutrients and vitamins to give your cells a helping hand in absorbing the nutrients. This, in turn, eliminated the toxins that are aging and drying your skin. The following is a list of the best foods for your skin and should be on your shopping list:

Red Peppers

Red peppers contain more than 9 times as much carotene and two times as much vitamin C than green peppers do, evidenced by their rich bright color. They also taste nicer! Red peppers contain folate, one of the best antioxidants for antiaging, along with vitamin A, which helps to stop the harmful UV rays from causing damage to your skin. They are also full of other antioxidants, which help to keep you healthy

Brown Rice

Brown rice is not only tastier and more textured than white rice, it also has more vitamin B1, which helps to regulate circulation, keeping it healthy. Good blood circulation helps to stop the loss of skin elasticity and also stops the skin from wrinkling. It has more fiber than any other type of rice because it has not been removed from its husk, making it one of the best foods for detoxing.

Berries

Berries may be small but they are capable of magic. One of the things they can do is prevent cellulite form forming by boosting your circulation and the flow of blood and lymph fluids. All of that stops your skin from dimpling in certain areas of the body and the antioxidants in the berries plump the cells out. This also stops your skin from looking worn out and tired.

Leafy Greens

Especially the darker ones. Leafy green vegetables are packed full of anti-oxidants, especially a coenzyme called Q10. No doubt you have heard of this, as it is an ingredient in many skin creams. However, you don't need to go to that expense when you can get the same coenzyme in its natural form by eating broccoli, kale and spinach, all of which are a lot cheaper than the latest anti-aging cream. Q10 helps cell to grow and, as we age, our bodies stop producing so much, thus needing a bit of a helping hand.

Quinoa

This is a pseudo-cereal that tastes similar to couscous or rice. It is one of the more expensive grains but is one of life's super foods, full of protein and great for anti-aging detoxification.

Lean Protein

If you tend to buy fatty cuts of meat, swap them out for lean cuts. Lean meat contains a lower level of saturated fat than regular cuts and this saves your body all the extra work of digesting and processing the excess. Lean proteins include chicken, oily fish and turkey, which all help to repair cells. Oily fish is good for boosting your collagen levels and is packed full of omega-3 essential fatty acids.

Cinnamon

Strangely, cinnamon stops the growth of bacteria and boosts brain function, as well helping to lower cholesterol, triglyceride and glucose levels. A good all-rounder, cinnamon cuts down damage to the cells, which helps your skin to stay looking younger.

Mediterranean Herbs

Herbs like oregano, parsley, rosemary and basil are all excellent ingredients for an anti-aging detox diet. Oregano is especially good as it has more than 20 times the potency of antioxidants than most other herbs.

Eggs

Eggs are a complete protein, which makes then an excellent choice for helping with the effects of aging. They contain vitamins A, B12, D and K as well as lutein, which also help to maintain the health of your eyes.

Walnuts and Cashews

Both of these contain copper, which, in low levels, can actually stop your hair from going grey prematurely. Copper helps the body to produce melanin, which is what gives your hair its color.

Fresh Fish

Fish is well known for its health benefits and you will always find them on any anti-aging detox diet. Fish like tilapia, salmon, sardines and trout contain very high levels of omega-3 and vitamins that help to keep you looking younger. Fish are also good for helping the cardiovascular system and promoting healthy eyes.

Herbal Teas

Herbal tea has long been known for helping to detox and improve skin health. Green tea in particular is one of the best but all herbal teas help to clean out your system, and push antioxidants through which help to fight off the damage done by free radicals. Tea is easily accepted by the body because it can extract the nutrients that help fight bacteria, heal up wounds, skin breaks, and cleanse those toxins right out.

Citrus Fruits

Citrus fruits such as lemons, limes, oranges and grapefruit can make you look younger because they are loaded with antioxidants. They help to flush the organs out, like your intestines, and will break down and remove bacteria and toxins. They also have high water content and, as you know by now, a detox is a waste of time if you don't keep your body hydrated. Citrus also has fat burning properties, thus making you look younger and helping you to burn off the unwanted pounds.

Pineapples

Pineapples are excellent parts of an anti-aging detox diet because they contain bromelain. This is a collection of enzymes that help to improve the health of your digestive system. The cleaner you colon is, the healthier you will feel and the younger you will look.

All of these foods will help to boost your immune system and keep it healthy, keeping you regular and reducing the chance of an infection. Tired and old looking skin happens because your skin is desperately trying to detox your body and this causes the spots, wrinkles and bags under the eyelids. Change your diet, change your life, it's a simple as that.

The next chapter is going to look at two different methods of detox – short and long-term, along with a few tips on how to detox safely.

How to Detox

Short-term

There are three main ways that you can do a short-term detox but, for all three methods, the real emphasis here is on short!

Fruit Detox

The fruit detox is a good way to detox without going hungry. Amongst the obvious health benefits of eating fruit, this also helps to increase your energy levels, lose weight, and could cut down on your chances of a stroke. You can do this eating just one type of fruit (make it your favorite one) or by eating a variety of different fruits. You must not go more than 7 days on a fruit detox diet!

For best results:

Choose citrus fruits such as oranges, grapefruits, lemons, tangerines, mandarins and limes. These contain excellent detoxifying properties and go well either on their own or combined with other fruits.

Try a grape detox. Grapes contain something called reservatrol (particularly red or black grapes) that can help to prevent blood clots and fight cancer and diabetes. They also contain high levels of vitamin C and potassium. For a maximum of 3-5 days, eat ONLY grapes and nothing else.

Liquid Detox

For 2-3 days eat nothing, just drink water, fruit juice, tea (green or black tea is best), vegetable juices and/or protein smoothies. These work by cutting down the amount of calories you are taking in and can help to flush out toxins from your body.

For best results:

Drink fruit and vegetable juices so that your body is receiving adequate nourishment, vitamins, and minerals. Make your own from fresh fruits and vegetables rather than drinking shop bought ones as these contain sugars and other ingredients you don't want.

If you choose a liquid detox, you will have to seriously rethink your diet if your goal is weight loss. Otherwise, as soon as you go back to a normal diet all the weight will go back on.

Fruit and Vegetable Detox

Instead of just fruits, eat a variety of vegetables as well for 7 days. Both contain minerals, vitamins and other vital nutrients that your body requires for optimum health. Eat a wide range to make sure you get all you need.

For best results:

- Eat beans, such as kidney and black beans, apples, blueberries, artichokes and soybeans for fiber
- Eat carrots, lima beans, cooked greens, sweet potatoes, ordinary potatoes, and bananas for potassium
- Eat strawberries, kiwi, cauliflower, tomato, kale, Brussels Sprouts, bell peppers, mango, and oranges for vitamin C
- Eat melons, cooked spinach, oranges, asparagus and black-eyed peas for folate
- Eat coconut, olives and avocadoes for good fats

Long-term

Change Your Diet

Swap processed foods for organic meat and organic produce. The fruit and vegetables you buy in a supermarket are grown using chemicals, herbicides, and pesticides while organic produce contains only natural fertilizers and pesticides. Organic meats are raised on natural grass and contain none of the chemicals, antibiotics, and growth hormones that are normally fed to animals.

For best results:

- Make sure everything you eat is organic – look for a green USDA Certified Organic Seal on packaging
- Only eat grass-fed animal products, such as meat, butter, milk, eggs, cheese, etc.
- Drink plenty of water, at least 2-4 liters every day. As well as keeping you hydrated, it flushes out the toxins from your kidneys. You don't have to drink plain water if you really can't face it, add fruit and vegetables to it – particularly citrus fruit as this helps to boost your fat-burning properties. Later, I will give you some recipes for flavored waters that will help you get through your day much easier
- Cut the alcohol. It has now been shown that alcohol is linked to cancer, so cut down to one glass a night, no more. Don't be tempted to cut it out all week and then binge on a Friday or Saturday night – that is far worse than drinking all week.
- Cut out sugar, which you will do if you remove processed foods from your diet anyway.

Detox Tips

- Try and detox with a friend for support
- Eat slowly. Chewing your food thoroughly helps with digestion and gives your body a chance to process all that it is receiving
- Don't forget the exercise. Stick to light exercise during a detox, such as Pilates or yoga.
- Rest up properly. Make sure you get sufficient sleep every night and add in afternoon naps if necessary.
- Go for a massage, it will help the toxins to come out of your

body much quicker

Warnings

Do not continue past the 7-10 days mark on a fasting detox. Long term fasting can do irreparable damage Research your detox diet thoroughly before undertaking it; speak to your doctor if necessary

Never fast to the point where you go lightheaded or actually faint. If you get to this stage, eat a slice of bread or a biscuit to bring your blood sugar levels up and drink a sports drink that contains electrolytes.

You might feel lethargic for the first couple of days – do not give up because this will pass. Just allow yourself that time to relax and don't do anything strenuous.

Never do a liquid fast for any more than three consecutive days.

In the next chapter, we are going to take a look at what you can and shouldn't eat on a detox diet. I will also be giving you a few ideas for water recipes as well.

Chapter 3:

What You Should and Shouldn't Consume on a Detox Cleanse

The whole idea of a detox cleanse is to cut out the rubbish, the foods and drinks that contributing to that buildup of toxins in your body. Now, it can be a little confusing when you start a detox cleanse diet, knowing what you can and can't eat. So, the following lists should help to clear up any confusion you may have.

Foods to Eat

Fruits:

- Any fruit, fresh or frozen
- Fruit juices – must be natural and unsweetened – if in doubt, make your own
- Unsweetened dried fruit in small amounts – raisins, cranberries, goji berries, etc.

Vegetables:

- Broccoli
- Cauliflower
- Spinach
- Kale
- Beet greens

- Collard greens
- Onions
- Broccoli sprouts
- Garlic
- Beets
- Artichokes
- Swiss chard
- Kelp
- Nori
- Wakame
- Tomatoes
- Bell peppers
- Egg plants
- Potatoes (depending on the type of detox you are on)
- Avoid corn, as it is highly acid forming

Grains/Starches:

- Brown rice
- Quinoa
- Millet
- Buckwheat
- Wild rice
- Amaranth
- Oats

Go for whole grains where possible but you can use products made from the above, such as bread, buckwheat noodles, rice crackers, or brown rice pasta

Beans/Legumes:

- Adzuki
- Lima
- Kidney
- Green
- Black-eyed peas
- Lentils
- Split peas – green or yellow

Nuts/Seeds:

- Cashews
- Walnuts
- Almonds
- Sunflower seeds
- Sesame seeds
- Pumpkin seeds
- Chia seeds
- Hemp nuts
- Hemp seeds
- Young coconut
- Nut butters made with any of the above
- Tahini

Avoid peanuts or peanut butters and go for nuts and seeds that are unsalted and raw

Oils:

- Olive oil – cold-pressed, extra virgin is best
- Flax oil
- Hemp oil
- Almond oil
- Chia oil
- Avocado oil
- Coconut oil

You can consume safflower, sunflower, and sesame oils in small amounts

Foods to Avoid

Dairy/Eggs:

- Eggs in all formats
- Cheese
- Milk
- Sour cream
- Cottage cheese
- Kefir
- Yogurt, including frozen

Wheat:

- Butter
- Ice cream

Any product that contains wheat in any format, including bread or pasta, unless made with approved ingredients

Sweeteners:

- Sugar – refined, white, brown, castor, etc.
- HFCS – High Fructose Corn Syrup
- Cane juice
- Any artificial sweetener
- Any liquid sweetener

If you must use sweetener of any kind, use a little natural honey

Gluten:

- Wheat
- Rye
- Barley
- Spelt
- Kamut
- Triticale
- Bran
- Couscous
- Farina

Soy Products:

- Milk
- Tofu
- Yogurt
- Sauce
- Protein powder
- Tempeh
- Caffeine:

- Coffee

- Tea

- Soft drinks

You can drink decaffeinated coffee and green tea

Detox Waters

If you find yourself unable to face drinking liters of plain water every day, fear not. There are plenty of ways to spice it up a bit and give it a better taste in ways that can speed up weight loss, and cleanse you much quicker. Give some of these a shot and see how much fun it can be to drink water:

Slim-Down

This is amazingly beneficial water, helping to flush toxins out of the body and fat as well. Cucumbers are natural diuretics, which stop the water retention, and citrus fruits help to flush toxins and burn fat:

- ½ gallon spring water

- ½ a medium grapefruit

- ½ a cucumber

- ½ a lemon

- ½ a lime

- Mint leaves

Slice all the fruit and the cucumber up and add it all to the water in a large jug. Add the mint leaves and refrigerate for a couple of hours before drinking. Aim for at least ½ a gallon per day.

Fruity Detox

As well as tasting fantastic in the summer months, the fruit in this contains vitamin A and vitamin E, which both aid the flushing of free radicals and toxins. Strawberries are excellent for anti-aging and help the skin to stay smooth and youthful looking as well as helping to fight off carcinogens.

- 2 liters spring water
- 2 large strawberries
- Two small to medium kiwis

Chop the fruit and add to the water. Refrigerate for a couple of hours before use and drink at least 2 liters daily. Increase the fruit to taste

Day Spa Apple Cinnamon

This wonderful water contains absolutely no calories, making it marvelous for slimming and for flushing out the toxins. And, it can help to boost your metabolism, thus speeding up the weight loss.

- 2 liters spring water
- 1 apple
- 2 or 3 cinnamon sticks

Slice the apple thinly and place it into a gallon pitcher with the cinnamon. Fill up the jug halfway with ice and then add the water. Leave it in the fridge for about an hour before serving. You can fill this jug up three or four times without changing the apple or cinnamon and you can increase the fruit or cinnamon if you want a stronger taste

New Year Detox

This is a great water to drink any time of the year, not just at New Year. It's a great tasting water to help boost your metabolism, burn off fate and get rid of the toxins in your body.

- 1 gallon spring water
- Handful of raspberries
- 1 grapefruit
- 1 cucumber

- 1 pear
- Couple of sprigs of mint

Slice the grapefruit, pear, and cucumber and add to the water with the raspberries and mint. Refrigerate for a couple of hours before drinking. For a zestier taste, add limes, lemons, cranberries and blueberries as well

Strawberry Vitamin

Strawberry infused water not only flushes toxins out, it also helps to keep your skin looking youthful as well as being full of anti-inflammatory properties and vitamins.

- 2 liters spring water
- 1 cup strawberries
- 2 cups watermelon
- 2 sprigs fresh rosemary
- Dash of coarse sea salt

Cube the watermelon and place in a large jug. Chop the strawberries in half and mix together with the rosemary. Add to the jug and pour water over. Stir, add the salt, and refrigerate for 2 hours. Stir again before drinking

Fat Burner

This is wonderful detox water that flushes out the toxins, helps you to burn fat, and drop those pounds as well. It's full of fiber, and the cinnamon helps to slow down your appetite.

- 12 oz. spring water
- 2 tbsp. apple cider vinegar
- 1 tbsp. fresh lemon juice
- 1 tsp ground cinnamon
- Half a medium apple

Put all the ingredients, except the apple, into the blender for 10 seconds. Slice the apple, add to the drink, and enjoy

Cucumber Lemon Detox

Lemon is an excellent cleanser and helps to boost the immune system while cucumber is a diuretic that helps you to keep hydrated and has anti-inflammatory properties. The mint is good for digestion and helps to sweeten the water.

- 8 cups spring water
- 1 medium cucumber
- 1 lemon
- 10 mint leaves

Cut the cucumber and lemon into wedges or slice it – your choice. Add to the water with the mint and leave in the fridge overnight before drinking

Aloe

We all know what aloe Vera is but how many of us realize what the benefits of it are? It is excellent for aiding digestion and circulation as well as getting rid of fatigue.

- 1 cup water
- 2 tbsp. fresh lemon juice
- 2 tbsp. aloe gel

To get the gel, split an aloe leaf down the center and scoop the gel out. Add to the other ingredients in the blender and blend for about 1 minute before drinking.

Lemon Ginger

Ginger is one of the best natural pain relievers there is. Adding it to the cleansing properties of lemon gives you a great water to start every day with as it works to flush toxins all day long.

- 12 oz. water
- ½" chunk of ginger root
- ½ lemon juiced

Add the lemon juice to the water and grate the ginger in. Stir well and drink straightaway. Make sure your water is at room temperature

Detox Smoothies and Juices

As well as waters, you also have the option or making raw fruit and vegetable juices and smoothies, if you fancy something a little more filling. Try the following:

Matcha Mango Pineapple Smoothie Ingredients

- 1 ¼ cups of Matcha Matsu green tea
- 1 scoop of protein powder
- 1 cup of fresh or frozen (defrosted) mango chunks
- 1 tbsp. 100% pineapple juice
- 1 cup fresh or frozen (defrosted) pineapple chunks
- ½ - 1 cup of water
- Honey to taste

Add all the ingredients into the blender and blend until smooth. The amount of water you use depends on how thick you want your smoothie to be.

Cranberry, Kale and Pomegranate Detox Juice Ingredients

- 4-6 kale leaves, large ones
- 1 cup of pomegranate arils – from a large pomegranate
- cup fresh or frozen (defrosted) cranberries
- 1 pear, cored
- About an inch of fresh ginger, peeled

- 6-12 mint leaves – optional
- Stevia to taste

Put the ingredients, one at a time, into the juicer, leaving the pomegranate seeds until last. Strain if you want to and serve straightaway

Detox Vegetable Juice Ingredients

- 1 or 2 large red peppers, deseeds ad sliced up
- 4 sliced tomatoes
- 3 carrots, cleaned, peeled and sliced
- 2 heads of romaine lettuce
- 1 celery bunch
- A large handful of cilantro
- 1 cucumber, peeled and chopped
- 2 peeled lemons
- About an inch of fresh ginger

Juice everything together and give it a good stir. This will make around 3 pints but you can refrigerate for up to 48 hours – don't forget to give it a good stir before serving.

Grapefruit-Cado Sunrise Smoothie Ingredients

- ½ fresh avocado
- ½ cup orange juice, fresh squeezed
- 1 up grapefruit juice, fresh squeezed
- 1 cup frozen strawberries
- ¾ cup frozen banana slices
- ¼ cup ice
- 1 tsp maple syrup to taste, optional

Blend all the ingredients together until smooth and serve. You can substitute fresh squeezed juice for 100% natural juices but using fresh fruit is better

Orange, Apple Carrot, Celery and Lime Juice Ingredients

- 2 apples, quartered
- 2 cleaned carrots, chopped
- 1 celery stalk. Chopped
- 4-5 limes

Juice everything together until you have the desired consistency and serve over ice. You can add crushed ice into the blender if you want

Blueberry Fruit Smoothie Ingredients

- ½ cup frozen blueberries
- ¼ cup cranberry juice, unsweetened
- ½ bananas

Blend the entire ingredient together until smooth and serve immediately

Veggie Pizza Juice Ingredients

- 4-5 Roma tomatoes
- 2 sweet bell peppers, 1 yellow, 1 orange
- 1/3 yellow onion
- A bunch of kale
- 1 peeled garlic clove
- 10-15 basil leaves
- Handful of raw cashew pieces

First, juice all of the ingredients, leaving out the cashew pieces. Then pour the juice into a blender, add the cashews and blend

Carrot and Beet Smoothie Ingredients

- 1 peeled carrot, sliced

- 1 peeled beet, sliced

- ½ cup grapes, red

- 1 peeled clementine, broken into segments

- A slice of peeled ginger

- ½ cup green tea

Put the carrot and beet slices into a steamer and cook gently for about 10-15 minutes, or until tender. Leave these to cool off. Now add all of the ingredients to the blender and blend until smooth

Detox Meals

You do not need to starve yourself on a detox diet, far from it so below, I have given you just three recipes that you can eat while detoxing. These are just to give you a basis to start from and a few ideas.

Breakfast

Blueberry-Coconut Bakes Oatmeal Ingredients
OATMEAL

- 1 ½ cups steel cut oats

- ½ tsp ground ginger

- ½ tsp sea salt, fine

- 1 tsp baking powder

- 4 cups vanilla almond milk, unsweetened

- 2 cups light coconut milk, unsweetened

- 1 ½ cups fresh blueberries

- ¼ cup dried unsweetened blueberries

- ¼ cup coconut flak, unsweetened

- Natural sweetener to taste

BLUEBERRY SAUCE

- 2 cups blueberries, fresh or frozen

OPTIONAL TOPPINGS

- Coconut flake

- Toasted nuts

- Extra blueberries, dried or fresh

- Whipped cream

- Coconut milk

Preparation OATMEAL

1 Preheat the oven to 350° F and put the oven rack in the center

2 Coat a baking dish 13 x 9 x 2 inch lightly with cooking spray

3 Mix all of the oatmeal ingredients together, adding the coconut and blueberries last

4 Sweeten to taste and bake for approximately 1 hour

5 When the time is out, take the oatmeal out of the over, although it won't look cooked. Leave it to cool and then refrigerate overnight to thicken up

BLUEBERRY SAUCE

1 Add a splash of water to the blueberries and heat over a medium high heat

2 When they start to sizzle, reduce the heat and cook for 5 minutes, or until they turn to a sauce-like consistency

3 Mash them against the side of the pan

4 Serve the oatmeal with a little coconut or almond milk and the blueberry sauce

5   Use any of the additional toppings if you want but don't overdo it

Lunch

Baked Sweet Potato and Greens Ingredients

- 2 sweet potatoes, pricked
- 1 tbsp. extra virgin olive oil
- 1 small onion, sliced thinly
- 1 bunch Swiss chard, stemmed and chopped
- Coarse salt
- 1 avocado pitted and sliced
- Cayenne pepper
- Lemon

Preparation

1   Preheat the oven to 400° F

2   Bake the potatoes for about 45 minutes, or until tender

3   Heat the oil in skillet and cook the onion until tender, around 6 minutes

4   Add the chard, stirring, and cook until it is bright green and has wilted, around 5 minutes

5   Season with the salt

6   Split the potatoes and top each one off with the greens and half the avocado

7   Season with salt, cayenne and a squeeze of lemon

Dinner

Chicken, Vegetable, Avocado and Rice Bowls Ingredients

CHICKEN

- 1 lb. chicken breast, boneless and skinless (if using skewers, cube it, if not, leave it whole)
- ¼ cup olive oil
- 4 garlic cloves, minced
- ½ tsp onion powder
- ½ tsp pepper
- ½ tsp cayenne
- ½ tsp smoked paprika
- ¼ cup chopped fresh parsley or 1 tbsp. dried
- ¼ cup chopped fresh basil or 1 tbsp. dried

RICE AND VEGETABLES

- 1 ½ cups rice, Basmati or jasmine
- 3 cups water
- 2 red peppers, quartered
- 1 zucchini, cut into ¼ inch rounds
- 1 tbsp. olive oil
- Salt and pepper to taste
- 2 avocadoes, pitted, peeled and mashed thoroughly
- Juice from 1 lemon
- ½ cup chopped fresh parsley
- 1 clove grated garlic
- 1 pint of halved grape or cherry tomatoes

- ¼ cup toasted walnuts
- ½ cup crumbled blue cheese – optional

Preparation

1   If you are using bamboo skewers, soak them for 30 minutes before you start grilling to stop them from charring

2   In a bowl, mix the garlic, olive oil, onion powder, paprika, cayenne, basil and parsley. Add in the chicken and toss to coat

3   Cover the bowl and refrigerate while you are making the rice

4   To make the rice, bring the water to a low boil and then drop the rice in. Stir it well, cover and reduce the heat as low as possible

5   Cook for 10 minutes, turn off the heat and leave the rice for a farther 20 minutes, covered – do not uncover at all, not even to take a look

6   After the 20 minutes is up, remove the lid and use a fork to fluff up the rice

7   Reheat the grill to medium high

8   Put the pepper and zucchini in a large Ziploc bag

9   Add a pinch of salt and pepper and 1 tbsp. of olive oil 10 Seal the bag and shake to coat the vegetables
11 Remove the chicken form the refrigerator

12 Either skewer it or leave it whole and cop it after grilling

13 Grill for about 3-4 minutes either side, turning it a couple of times until thoroughly cooked and with light char marks across it

14 At the same time, grill the zucchini, about 4 minutes either side and the peppers for 5 minutes 15 Remove the food from the grill and leave for 5 minutes to cool down

16 Slice the peppers into strips and cut whole chicken breast into

cubes (if you are not skewering it)

17 Put the avocado mash into a bowl, add the garlic, parsley, salt, pepper and lemon juice to taste, stirring well

18 Divide the rice over 4 serving bowls

19 Top each one with chicken, pepper and zucchini (or a couple of skewers)

20 Add a large spoon of the avocado mix and top off with tomatoes and walnuts, sprinkling blue cheese over if you want to

21 Serve immediately

15 Detox Salads

Salads do not need to be boring! Most people turn their noses up at salad because they think only of the basics, like lettuce, tomato and cucumber. While these do make a very nice salad, there are tons of other ingredients that you can add. Most salads have a detox effect on the body but the ones I am going to tell you about are especially detoxifying and will help to clean your system out a bit.

A detox salad is nothing more than a bunch of ingredients that all have a detox effect. A lot of the time, we chop these ingredients up finely, to allow for easier chewing and digestion. A lot of these ingredients are high in fiber, which helps your digestive system to work properly, and some are designed to clean the kidneys and the liver. Yet others will help to stock up your body with the nutrients and vitamins it so badly needs. Each of these salads is different, and each has its own effect on your body. I am not giving you exact recipes here, just the ingredients – use them in the quantities that you want!

1. Rainbow Salad and Roast Squash

This is a very pretty salad but, aside from that, it is highly beneficial to the body. The roast squash blends very well

with the rest of the ingredients to provide a filling and satisfying salad that will keep you full for some time. Simple slice and deseed a small squash, leaving the skin on. Season with salt and pepper before roasting. Steam some broccoli florets. Mix tender greens, diced red onion, sliced red cabbage, radishes and pumpkin seeds together in a bowl. Serve topped with the roast squash and broccoli and the (healthy) dressing of your choice for a salad that is full of fiber.

2. Simple Detox Salad

While this might look like a basic salad, it is much more. The ingredients will be working hard to deliver fiber, nutrients and vitamins, as well as healthy fats, antioxidants and potassium, all designed to help the body rid itself of toxins. Simply take a bunch of kale that has been de-stemmed and chopped up and add it to red cabbage, carrots, black beans, mushrooms, roasted beets, red peppers, sunflower seeds and roasted Brussels sprouts. Top off with half an avocado.

3. Winter Detox Salad

So many people think salads are just for warmer weather and detoxing is only for the spring months but this salad is perfect for a cold gray winter's day. In the winter, our bodies tend to retain more of what we eat and we need to get that digestive system moving so you are not building up a body full of toxins. That is exactly what this salad is for. Chop up a couple of medium sized rutabaga heads and add grated carrot, pomegranate seed, pine nuts and pink peppers. Make a dressing from olive oil, fresh lemon juice and pink Himalayan salt and toss the salad in it.

4. Quinoa, Almond and Apple

You do not need to stick to vegetables for a perfect salad. Instead, fruits, nuts and grains can do just as good a job of cleansing your body. Quinoa is filling; apple is full of nutrients, as well as being a superfood as are the almonds. Cook the quinoa and allow to cool. Mix with toasted chopped almonds, diced apple, cranberries and scallions for a tasty healthy salad.

5. Cauliflower and Broccoli Detox Salad

Both of these vegetables are members of the cruciferous family and, while they taste completely different, the benefits they give you are somewhat similar. Both contain heaps of vitamins and nutrients and, with the addition of the carrots and the sunflower seeds give you a complete body cleanse. Mix steamed broccoli and cauliflower florets with shredded carrot, sunflower seeds, currants, raisins and fresh parsley. Season with a little salt and lots of pepper, drizzle lemon juice over and, if you can get them, or indeed want them, add a sprinkling of kelp granules.

6. Shredded Vegetable Salad

The idea behind shredding everything is that it makes it easier to chew and is easier on the digestive system too. You can make up a big bath of this on and eat it for a few days but do drizzle lemon juice and olive oil over it to preserve it for longer. Use your food processor to shred carrots, and then chop the cauliflower, kale, broccoli and parsley into very small chunks. Toss together with sunflower seeds and raisins and dress with lemon juice and olive oil.

7. Gluten-Free

Not everyone can eat foods that contain gluten so you need to choose detox foods that keep you to your gluten-free lifestyle. Most of the salads on this list are actually gluten-free but sometimes there is the odd ingredient that contains it. And, because this salad contains no animal byproducts, it's also a great one for vegans. Process broccoli and cauliflower into very small pieces and do the same with a carrot. Mix together in a bowl and add in fine chopped kale, sunflower seeds, chopped parsley, sliced almonds, currants and blueberries. Mix lemon juice, mild vinegar and maple syrup for a dressing and add kelp powder if you want to.

8. Kale Salad

All too often, we are told we must eat more kale but there are only so many ways you can eat it. As well as mixing it in green smoothies, you can also add it to this tasty salad. The addition of cucumber helps with hydration as well as balancing the kale taste out as well. Avocado gives you a healthy dose of the good fats, making it a fully cleansing super-salad. Mix sliced kale and chopped scallions with shelled edamame and diced cucumber. Dice the avocado and toss it in lemon juice before adding it to the salad. Make a dressing from olive oil, lemon zest, mirin, cayenne, ginger and salt and drizzle over the salad. Toss well and top off with pinenuts or sunflower seeds.

9. Asparagus and Tomato Salad

One common misconception about salads is that they have to have lots of different ingredients to actually be classed as a salad. Some of the best salads have only a couple of ingredients that go well together, Asparagus and tomatoes are two of those foods, both providing nutritious and cleansing benefits to the body. Thinly slice a bunch of raw asparagus and mix it with halved cherry tomatoes. Make a dressing from lemon juice, vinegar, salt and pepper and toss the asparagus and tomatoes in it. You can add a sprinkling of shaved parmesan cheese as well if you want it.

10. Roasted Beets and Pumpkin Seeds

Roasted beets are a fantastic detox food – but only if you use raw beets that you cook, NOT pickled ones. The addition of pumpkin seeds and greens completes this bountiful salad full of fiber and nutrition, as well as antioxidants. Cook and cool the beetroots or buy them ready cooked. Cut into cubes. Put mesclun greens, or whichever you prefer, into a bowl and top with the beet cubes and pumpkin seeds. You can add crumbled goats cheese if you want but it isn't a highly detoxifying food. Drizzle a dressing made from olive oil and balsamic vinegar over the salad and enjoy – both you and your liver!

11. Everyday Detox Salad

You don't have to make detoxing a one-off thing; you can give your body exactly what it needs every single day. This salad combines miso and carrot for a tasty dressing that will make you crave this over and over again. The salad is based on that healthy superfood spinach with cucumbers and tomatoes providing a flavorsome, nutrient dense salad. To make this salad, chop up a spinach, red onion, cherry tomatoes, cucumbers, and cilantro and mix it all together in a bowl. Make the dressing from chopped carrots and shallots, grated ginger, white miso paste rice vinegar. Sesame oil, water and vegetable or olive oil – just mix it all up and toss your salad in it.

12. The Happy Salad

The name really does say it all here – your body will be over the moon if you give it this salad on a regular basis and you will be giving it exactly what it needs in terms of nutrition. The ingredients in this salad ensure that you will have more energy and your elimination system will be more regular, making you feel good in body and mind. Chop carrots, green cabbage, green onions and steamed broccoli. Make a dressing from maple syrup, lemon zest, minced garlic, minced or grated ginger and add a little salt and pepper. Toss your salad in it and sprinkle a few sunflower seed kernels over the top – as many as you want really.

13. The Day after Detox Salad

We all go through days and nights of heavy celebration – weddings, birthdays, holiday season, etc. – and this salad is designed for the day after a bag over indulgence. It is standard as far as detox salads go but it does have one ingredient that is scientifically proven to provide your intestines with healthy flora, thus helping your digestive system to get moving and your elimination system to work properly. You need some roughly chopped carrots. Steamed broccoli chopped up. Grape tomatoes, sunflower seeds, all mixed and tossed in a dressing made from grapeseed oil, apple cider vinegar, nutritional yeast, lemon juice, salt and pepper. Leave it chilling in the refrigerator for about 30 minutes before you eat it.

14. Citrus, Seeds and Greens Salad

Citrus fruits are known for their naturally cleansing properties, which makes them the perfect addition to any detox diet. Every ingredient in this salad will hit your body with bolts of goodness and nutrition. The contrast between the tart citrus, the bitter greens and the crunchy nuts will be an assault on your taste buds, one that you will keep going back for time and time again. And if you really don't like the taste of greens then this is the perfect salad for you – you get a healthy serving of them with their taste disguised almost completely by the citrus.

You need a big bunch of greens – lettuce, spinach, arugula, rocket, etc. – a grapefruit, an orange, a lemon, sunflower seeds and pumpkin seeds. Mix it altogether, drizzle a little olive oil over the top, season with salt and pepper and enjoy.

15. Detox Slaw

This is a slaw that has delusions of being a salad or it could be a salad that thinks it might be a slaw. Whichever way it is, you can be sure you are getting a healthy dose of vegetables, especially cabbage. Cabbage is a wonderful superfood and you really should eat more of it. You don't need to shred this as much as you would a normal slaw ether so your teeth can get a bit of exercise too.

You will need red and green cabbage, carrots, fresh ginger, shelled edamame, radishes, water, salt, garlic, sherry vinegar, a shallot, olive oil and a lime. Shred the vegetables and mix them together. Then toss them in a dressing made from radish, carrot, miso paste, water, vinegar, ginger, lime and olive oil. Add a bit of garlic for good measure.

18 Teas for a Daily Detox Cleanse

Tea drinking may be something of a British custom but anyone can enjoy a daily cup of cleansing tea. Detox teas are soothing, and if you drink a different one off this list every day, you will be getting the full range of cleansing and detoxifying effects. These teas are idea for filling you with healthy nutrients and antioxidants at a cost that any pocket can afford. All of these teas can be bought from health stores, pharmacies or supermarkets. Or, if you choose, you can make your own.

1. Burdock Root Tea

Burdock is one of the little-know herbs that is full of detoxifying properties. As well as helping to purify the blood, it can strengthen your immune system. It is perfect for the liver and for the digestive system, which are the two main detox paths that the human body has. If your liver is functioning well, you will have less toxins in your blood and if your digestive system is working to keep you regular, the toxins won't have a chance to build up.

2. Cayenne Pepper Tea

It is only recently that cayenne pepper has become popular for its health benefits and more people are starting to use it to spice up their meals. However, it can also be brewed up as a tea and, in this format, it will give you a healthy dose of energy while cleansing your body. If you don't like it too spicy, add a slice of lemon. This will take the edge off the spice, cleanse the palate and help your digestive system get moving.

3. Chicory Tea

Chicory tea is fantastic for detoxing the body and it can also help to give your metabolism a huge boost, giving you a double dose of goodness. Chicory is good for getting the digestive juices revved up before you eat, making it easier to digest your food. If you choose to make this yourself use dried chicory as it contains more taste, more of the essence and plenty of vitamins.

4. Cilantro Tea

Most people add cilantro to their food to provide a strong taste but you can make a perfectly good detox tea from it as well. Cilantro is fast becoming one of the most popular herbs that helps enormously with the digestive system. It can help your body to better process foods by breaking them down more efficiently and making use of more of the nutrients, before it effective eliminates what isn't needed.

5. Dandelion tea

Dandelions are always seen as a bad weed in the garden but they are one of the most purifying "weeds" ever grown. Scientific research has shown that dandelion increases the levels of a particular enzyme that is known for being a detoxifying enzyme. They have also been known to remove toxins that may cause cancer from the body as well, making it extremely worthwhile to drink.

6. Fenugreek Tea

Fenugreek is known for helping with the digestion and can be very helpful whenever you feel as though your digestive system has sowed right down. For some people who constantly feel bloated or suffer with indigestion, this can be a daily drink. Other might find it beneficial to drink once a week. There are also some other benefits to drinking fenugreek tea; it can lower your blood pressure and help to reduce inflammation in the body.

7. Garlic Tea

Everyone should already know of the massive benefits that garlic provides and drinking it made into a tea is hugely cleansing. This is because it is full of vitamins and sulfur which is one of the most effective ingredients for detoxifying the body.

8. Ginger Tea

Ginger is another food that is excellent for cleansing the body and it tastes lovely brewed up as a tea. It is very gentle on your body, despite the tartness it has and that makes it perfect for daily use. Not only is it good at helping with detoxification, it can also be used as warming drink or as a pick-me-up and a boost to energy levels.

9. Green Tea

Green tea has amazing benefits and is one of the most widely written about teas. It has been scientifically proven that drinking one cup of green tea every day will improve your health no end. It is packed full of antioxidants that fight against free radicals and tons of other toxins and it has one other added benefit – the removal of all those toxins helps you to shed weight without even trying.

10. Guduchi Tea

You may not have heard of this herb but you should give it a go. It has long been used in many parts of the world for its restorative properties and it contains a long list of benefits. Those benefits include improving your skin, ridding the body of toxins and helping with the digestive system, amongst many others and this is all because it assist the organs to work the way they should do.

11. Gymnema Sylvestre Tea

This is a Chinese herb that has major effects on glucose. We all know that too much blood sugar can be extremely toxic and this tea helps to regulate that as well as helping your body to function properly. It can help with the liver and the digestive system so it is definitely one to try.

12. Manjistha Tea

The skin is the single largest organ of the human body and that makes it one of the biggest ways to remove toxins. If your skin is not getting the right nutrients and the support that it needs, it can't help in the detox process. Manjistha is a plant that is full of medicinal properties that work well when it is drunk. It is also an excellent choice for women who suffer with bad menstrual problems, because of the effect it has on helping to purify the blood.

13. Milk Thistle Tea

Milk thistle contains huge benefits for the liver, which is the focal point for most of the other organs in the body. This means that when your liver is functioning properly, neither are your other organs. Your liver should be the main focus of any detox plan you undertake and milk thistle is perfect for that. It is also good for the digestive system, thus doubling the detox effect.

14. Neem Tea

Neem is an herb that is highly popular in India and it can drunk as a tea to ward off loads of different diseases and conditions. It helps the liver to perform better and is full of minerals and vitamins that the body needs on a daily basis.

15. Red Clover Tea

Red clover is packed full of antioxidants which help the body to fight off free radicals that we consume with our food and breather in from our environment. Daily boosts of these antioxidants is vital to stop the free radicals from accumulating in the body. Without any defense mechanism in pace, those free radicals can cause all sorts of conditions that you really don't want.

16. Triphala Tea

Triphala is used to stimulate the bowels and is often used as a way of treating constipation. The toxins that build up in your body have to be eliminated somehow and if the colon and bowels are not working like they should, the toxins will simply build up and end up being reintroduced back into your body. Triphala tea, drunk daily, or even a couple of times a week will stop this from happening.

17. Turmeric Tea

Many people use turmeric as a way of spicing up a meal but it can also be made into a tea very easily. Turmeric is one of the most potent natural anti-inflammatories that can help with all sorts of problems caused by inflammation. It can also help the liver and kick start the gallbladder into producing bile, which is needed to help break the toxins down and get them out of your body. Taken on a daily basis, turmeric is a great way to get your digestive system working optimally.

18. Wormwood Tea

Wormwood is an herb that helps the bile to get out of the liver and out of your body, which is useful to stop toxic buildups from stagnating in the body. Wormwood has a purging effect and is perfect as a daily tea to ensure that your body is making sufficient bile and that it is getting through your system, as it should.

10 Cleansing and Revitalizing Soups

Detox soups contain many of the best and healthiest ingredients there are and bring them altogether in one delicious pot. Mostly you will need to blend or puree the vegetables or very finely chop them for best results. Doing this makes it easier on your body to digest them and that means your body gets to absorb more of the nutrients. The best bit about these soups is that they all taste beautiful while giving you a good dose of detoxifying minerals and vitamins.

Hot and Sour Soup – Vegetarian

This soup uses apple cider vinegar to give it the sour taste. Apple cider vinegar is widely known for its qualities in helping to replenish digestive flora. Use a mixed mushroom pack or use shitake or reishi mushrooms, both known for having detoxifying properties.

Ingredients:

- 1 oz. mixed dried mushrooms
- 8 cups water
- 3 tbsp. sherry wine for cooking
- ¼ cup apple cider vinegar
- 2 tbsp. soy sauce
- 1 ½ tsp kosher salt
- 1 tbsp. grated ginger

- 1 lb. tofu, extra firm, cut into cubes of ½ inch
- 2 tbsp. cornstarch
- 2 lightly beaten eggs
- 6 trimmed and sliced scallions
- ¼ tsp white pepper
- Pure sesame oil for serving

Instructions:

- Put the mushrooms into a bowl containing 2 cups of boiling water. Cover and leave for at least 30 minutes to rehydrate
- Strain the mushrooms, retaining the water for the soup
- Slice them thinly
- Add the remaining 6 cups of water to the mushroom liquid in a soup pot and then add the mushrooms
- Bring to the boil and add the vinegar, sherry, salt, soy sauce, tofu and ginger. Turn the heat down and simmer for 10 minutes, uncovered
- Take about ¾ a cup from the broth and mix the cornstarch in until it has dissolved
- Pour back into the soup, stirring to ensure it is distributed – the soup should slightly thicken
- Keep stirring and pour the eggs into the soup
- Add the pepper and scallions and cook for another couple of minutes
- Serve with a drizzle of the sesame oil

Spicy Tender Green Soup

With celery as a base, you can't go wrong with this soup. Celery is a wonderfully cleansing vegetable that we really don't eat enough of but this soup makes it easy to get a real dose of vitamins and nutrients to help cleanse your body and fill you up with fiber.

Ingredients – serves 2

- 4 stalks celery
- 1 yellow onion
- 1 bell pepper – green
- 5 generous handfuls of spinach
- 2 cloves garlic
- ½ tsp cardamom
- ½ tsp ground ginger
- ½ tsp ground cumin
- 1 tsp ground mint
- 1 liter water
- Fresh ground black pepper and seas salt for seasoning
- Optional – coconut milk or cream

Instructions:

- Bring the water to a boil and add sea salt to taste
- Chop up the celery, pepper, onion and spinach and add them to the water
- Cover the pot and cook over a medium heat for about 15 minutes or until the vegetables have softened up
- Turn the heat off and add the whole garlic cloves.

- Blend the soup and serve with black pepper and cream or coconut milk if desired

Radish and Leek Soup

The humble radish gets nowhere near the respect it deserves but by adding it to this soup with leeks, you get a double nutritious punch. Potato gives the soup some texture and sea kelp finishes it off nicely. Radishes have a subtle taste when cooked if you do not use too many and are known as a cancer fighting food and a blood purifier.

Ingredients:

- ¾ lb. radishes, cut in half
- 3 Yukon potatoes, peeled and cut into cubes
- 2 whole trimmed leeks
- 32 oz. chicken broth
- 1-2 tsp sea kelp seasoning
- 2 tbsp. butter
- 1 cup milk, whole
- Salt and pepper for seasoning

Instructions:

- Separate the leek tops and slice them up the stalk. Wash the leaves well and set to one side
- Put the butter in a pot and turn the heat up. Add the radishes, potatoes and sea kelp seasoning
- Mix well and then add the chicken broth. Stand the leek leaves up in the pot and bring the soup to a boil before reducing the heat to a simmer
- Leave to simmer for 60 minutes or until the vegetables have

softened. Remove the leek tops and blend the soup in a blender

- Add the milk, blend again, serve with salt, and pepper to taste.

Lentil, Sweet Potato and Kale Stew

One of the best ways to get a detox soup or stew is to use foods together that are superfoods on their own. Lentils are great for keeping the digestive system on the move and the kale is just one of the best superfoods you could ever eat, being full of nutrients and antioxidants. The sweet potatoes add extra fiber and a broad range of nutrients.

Ingredients:

- 1 can diced tomatoes, low sodium variety
- 2 cups of chicken or vegetable broth, low sodium
- 1 cup dried green lentils
- 1 bell pepper, green or red, diced
- 1 tbsp. curry powder
- Pinch of cumin or garam masala (optional
- 3 cloves of garlic
- 1 bunch coarsely chopped kale
- 2 cups if water
- 1 small zucchini, diced (optional)

Instructions

- Sauté the onions in a little olive oil
- After 3 minutes, add the potatoes, curry powder and garlic
- Sauté for 5 minutes until all the vegetables are tender
- Add the tomatoes, broth, lentils and water
- Simmer for 45 minutes over a low heat or until the lentils

have gone tender

- Add the pepper and kale right at the end and cook for 10 more minutes

- Serve and enjoy

Healthy Detox Soup

When you have kale in your kitchen, you can add it to any soup to turn it into a detox soup. In this soup there are lots more vegetables that support the kale and provide a broad spectrum of minerals, vitamins and other nutrients. The citrus from the lemon provides a cleansing benefit and the pepper helps the body to absorb the nutrients from the rest of the vegetables

Ingredients:

- 2 medium leeks, halved, cleaned and chopped into small chunks
- 4 cloves garlic, crushed to a paste
- 1 serrano pepper, thinly sliced with half of the seeds taken out
- 4 carrots, cleaned and cut into chunks – leave the skins on
- 4 stalks celery, cut into chunks
- 3 small rutabagas, peeled and medium diced
- 3 small diced zucchini
- 8 cups water
- 3 Roma tomatoes, diced with the skin and the seeds
- 2 cups Pint beans
- 2 bunches thin sliced kale
- Sale and fresh cracked black pepper for seasoning
- Juice from ½ lemon

Instructions

- Heat up a large pot over a medium heat and then add the garlic, serrano pepper and leeks

- Sweat the vegetables on a low heat for 5 minutes, stirring regularly

- Add the rutabaga, celery and carrots and cook for a further 3 minutes

- Add the beans, water and tomatoes and simmer on a low heat for 30 minutes or more – the longer you leave it, the better the flavor

- About 15 minutes before you are due to serve it, add the zucchini and kale

- Cook for 5 minutes before stirring n the lemon juice

- Season with the salt and pepper and serve hot.

Potassium Balancing Soup

Potassium is a vital nutrient that many of us forget about. Luckily, if your levs are too low it is very easy to fix, simply by eating more foods that are rich in the nutrient. This soup is designed to boost your potassium intake in more than one way. The kale has 329 milligrams of potassium per cup and carrots are not much less than that. The avocado is optional but it too contains a whole load of potassium, more than there is in one banana, as well as containing a whole bunch of other nutrients and healthy fats.

Ingredients:

- 3 large or 4 medium zucchini
- 4-6 large kale leaves
- 3-4 onions – green or spring
- 2 carrots

- 3 stalks of celery – if you are on a very low sodium diet leave these out.

- 1 lb. fresh green beans

- Bunch of fresh parsley

- Handful of cilantro (coriander)

- 3 tomatoes or a can of chopped tomatoes, low sodium variety

- 3 cloves of garlic

- 3 tbsp. tamari – omit if you are on a low sodium or a migraine diet

- 2 tbsp. seaweed flakes or use 1-2 sheets of nori, toasted and crumbled up – not if you are on a migraine diet

- 2 tbsp. amaranth or teff seeds – optional

- 1 sliced avocado

Instructions

- Wash the vegetables and put ach one through your food processor, chopping finely, one vegetable type at a time – make sure you leave the stems on the kale as this is where the potassium is

- Keep a bit of parsley back for garnishing

- Add each chopped vegetable to a heavy stock pot

- When the last one is in, add 1 liter of filtered or spring water

- Add the tamari, seaweed and teff or amaranth seeds, stirring well

- Bring up to a gentle boil, reduce the heat, cover and simmer for 30 minutes before serving

Kale and Lentil Soup

While kale and lentils are the named vegetables in this soup, there are loads of other that are great for your detox plan. If you just ate kale on its own, your body would be getting a detox; add the lentils and you get extra fiber, boosting your digestive system. The addition of parsley, garlic and carrots makes this a truly cleansing and highly nutritional soup.

Ingredients

- 8 cups of vegetable broth
- 1 ½ cups rinsed red lentils
- 2 carrots, cleaned and chopped
- 2 diced onions
- 1 bunch of kale, de-stemmed and roughly chopped
- 1 clove of garlic
- ¼ tsp red pepper flakes – optional
- 1 tbsp. chopped parsley – chop first and then measure
- Zest from ½ a lemon

Instructions

- Put the vegetable broth into a large saucepan with the carrots, lentils, garlic, onions and kale
- Bring up to the boil and cook for about 15 or 20 minutes, until the lentils are tender
- Add the red pepper flakes if using, the zest and parley
- Stir well and serve hot

Broccoli and Pea Pot

You cannot go wrong if you eat broccoli and adding it to any dish turns that dish into a detox recipe. Each serving of this soup contains ¼ lb. of broccoli and the lentils provide a good boost of fiber as well as protein.

The rest of the ingredients simply reinforce this thick soup as perfect for detoxing.

Ingredients

- 1 tbsp. olive oil
- ¼ cup green onions, chopped
- 1 finely chopped shallot
- 1 lb. of broccoli florets
- 1 tbsp. fresh thyme leaves
- ¼ tsp salt
- ½ tsp ground black pepper
- 3 cups of vegetable broth – homemade is best if you have some
- ¾ cup peas, frozen and thawed out is fine
- ¾ cup cooked brown or green lentils
- 1-2 cups of fresh spinach, de-stemmed and cleaned, torn into small chunks

Instructions

- Heat up a little oil in a heavy pan until it is hot and then add the shallots and green onion
- Cook for about 3-5 minutes, stirring constantly
- Add in the broccoli, salt, pepper and thyme – sauté for about 5 minutes
- Add the broth and bring it up to the boil
- Add in the peas and the lentils and then cook for another 5-10 minutes, or until the vegetables have softened to tender
- Cool it slightly and then add the spinach

- Separating the soup into smaller batches, puree it in a blender until it is smooth and creamy

- Put back in the pot and heat on a low heat until hot

- Add salt and pepper to taste and serve hot

Detox Green Machine Soup

Spinach makes an appearance in this recipe. It is one of the most nutrition dense foods available but it should really be combined with other ingredients, otherwise your soup will end tasting only of spinach. Green beans, zucchini and celery provide a wonderful taste along with a whole bunch of vitamins and minerals why the garlic, parsley and basil ensure that you will keep returning to the pot time after time for more of this detoxifying soup.

Ingredients

- 1 lb. green beans, fresh or frozen and thawed will do well

- 8 sticks of celery

- 4 lb. zucchini

- 2 generous bunches of spinach

- 1 whole yellow onion

- 5 cloves of garlic

- 1 bunch of parsley

- 1 bunch of basil

Instructions

- Put the green beans, the celery and the zucchini into a steamer and steam for about 15 minutes, or until they are very soft. Do not boil as you will lose most of the nutrients

- Add the garlic, onion and spinach to the steamer. Cook for a further 5 minutes

- If you want your soup to be thick drain off the excess water.

- Add in the parley and the basil and puree the soup until it is smooth

- Add salt and pepper to taste and serve hot

Apple and Roast Butternut Squash Soup

Roasting up a butternut squash is time consuming but it is really worthwhile. Let's face it, store bought butternut soup does not cut the mustard when it comes to taste; you simply can't beat a homemade version. Combined with the humble superfood, the apple you create a soup that is wonderful for the body. And add in those spices and you have a truly cleansing soup.

Ingredients

- 2-3 lb. of butternut squash, cut into 1 inch cubes

- 4 large apple, sweet ones like a Honeycrisp or a Gala, cut into 1 inch cubes

- 4 stalks of celery, chopped into 2 inch pieces

- 8 oz. mushrooms, halved

- 1 large onion cut into quarters

- ¼ cup of olive oil, a good quality one

- 4 cups of chicken or vegetable broth, low sodium

- 1 cup apple juice

- 2 tsp salt plus a little extra for taste

- 1 tsp black pepper pus a bit extra for taste

- ½ tsp nutmeg

- 1 tsp cinnamon

- ½ tsp red pepper flakes – optional if you want a bit of an extra kick to the soup

- Pumpkin seeds for garnish – optional

Instructions

- Preheat the oven to 425° F or 220° C

- Mix the butternut squash cubes with the onion and about a eighth of a cup of good quality olive oil

- Star to coat the butternut thoroughly

- Put the onion and butternut into a large roasting tin, together with the oil and back for about 30-40 minutes, or until the squash is tender to put a fork through

- Mix the apples with the mushrooms and the rest of the oil

- Put these into another roasting tin and bake until soft and fragrant, about 15-20 minutes

- Pour the broth into a large soup pan; add the apple juice and all of the roasted vegetables. Stir well

- Use an immersion blender to puree the vegetables and liquid in the pot. Alternatively, you can puree the vegetables in your blender first, along with the liquid; although you may need to do this is batches.

- If the consistency is too thick, add a little more broth or water.

- Simmer over a low-medium heat until hot

- Season with the spices, stirring them in well to distribute

- Serve hot garnished with the pumpkin seeds or, if you prefer a little fresh parsley or thyme and a swirl of cream.

Chapter 4:

7 Steps to Detox Your Body From Sugar

You might not think of sugar as something that you need to detox from but there are a couple of factors that influence this – the first is that sugar is not natural and the second is that human beings have only really been eating sugar for a relatively short period of time. This should make you realize that it is something that should only be eaten in small quantities yet, much of what you eat has sugar in it. In fact, many of our foods are loaded with sugar and it isn't really your fault that you eat too much of it. Sugar is a highly addictive substance but there is something you can do – first, become consciously aware of how much sugar you are eating and second, do something about purging your body of the sugar and your cravings for it. The following seven steps are designed to help your body and mind detox from the sugar monster.

Step 1 – Wean yourself off gradually or go cold turkey – your choice

You are the only person that truly knows you so only you can decide whether to cut sugar from your life gradually or in one hit. To be fair, both ways can be very successful but only if they are applied to right personality. Some people will respond best to a gradual reduction, while others respond better to a complete change. If you are at all unsure which one is you, start by weaning yourself off it gradually and see how you go. However you do it, this process is going to take time – there is no quick way to condition yourself not to crave sugar and all things that are sweet and it is going to be a tough habit to break.

Step 2 – Do a Candida Cleanse

Candida is a nasty beast that feeds on the sugar you eat. When you stop feeding it, it causes you to create more. Candida is also responsible for making you want foods that are high in these tasty carbohydrates that are so bad for you, like pasta and bread. These foods all add to your weight and many of them contain sugar. There are lots of candida cleanses that you can do, each with its own method. One thing I can tell you – by cutting sugar out, you will NOT rid your body of candida so it is a good idea to do a cleanse anyway. This is the only way to kill off the fungus that cause you to crave the sugar in the first place.

Step 3 – Change to a natural form of sugar.

One part of a sugar detox is to get your body used to eating natural forms of sugar and not the manmade poison that has only been in our lives for a short time. Today's sugar has been highly refined and is engineered to make it cheap. There is a word of difference between organic raw honey and High Fructose Corn Syrup (HFCS) and the sooner you can flush out the refined sugar and move to natural forms, the better you will feel. Do be careful how much you eat though, because even natural sugars can give you a taste for the sweet stuff.

Step 4 – Exercise

Exercising more will hasten up the process of getting rid of these cravings. As well as keeping you busy and out of temptations way, exercise also provides a natural high. This high can easily replace the high that sugar gives you. It has been proven that, when you are looking to get rid of a toxic bad habit, the easiest way is to replace that with something else that gives you the same or better rewards. Exercise is a fantastic option because it occupies your mind, makes you feel better, gives you more energy and helps you to work off the pounds that the sugar has accumulated.

Step 5 – Check your food labels properly

Sugar is not always the easiest ingredient to find on a food label so what you need to do is learn all the different terms for the many different sugars in your foods. Quite apart from trying to spot the word "sugar", you should also look for anything that is syrup as these are usually made from sugar. Sweetener is another common word and you should also be looking for words like Maltose, Dextrose, lactose, Dextrin and Fructose. HCFS is another one you may see. The best thing to do is look at the total sugar content on the nutrition label if there is one. If sugar is listed, look through the ingredients to see which types. Some people just give up eating prepackaged and processed foods altogether because virtually all of them include some kind of sugar.

Step 6 – Don't make the mistake of switching sugar for an artificial sweetener

You can't get the best of your addiction to sugar by using artificial sweeteners because they are no better. Instead of making you feel better, all you are doing is switching sugar for a bunch of unknown chemicals that can actually cause worse health problems than sugar can. While many of these sweeteners may provide a sweet taste without actually being sugar, they are not very widely studies and what we do know about them is not good. If you must use one, go for something like Stevia or truvia because these are pure natural sugars that do not contain the chemicals.

Step 7 – Stay diligent

The single biggest setback you will face when you detox your body from sugar is a relapse. It may be just one soda or just one cookie but that can undo all the work you have done and set you back in your old ways. It never is just one, that is the nature of addiction and sugar is one of the most addictive substances in the food world. If you really feel that you are going to struggle, try cutting back for a month or so until you have more control over your cravings. If you do relapse, start again and do not get frustrated – that will just lead to you throwing the towel in.

Detox Desserts

Just so you don't think you are missing out altogether, there are some great desserts you can eat on a detox plan that use natural forms of sugar and taste fantastic.

Chia Pudding Ingredients

- 1 cup of regular milk, almond milk or coconut milk – unsweetened variety

- 1 tbsp. raw organic honey

- 2 tbsp. whole chia seeds

Instructions

- Put all the ingredients into a bowl and mix together thoroughly

- Leave to sit for about 2 minutes and then mix again so the mixture doesn't go lumpy

- If you end up using sweetened milk, do not use the honey as well

Detox Cookies Ingredients

- 3 bananas, very ripe

- ½ cup of unsweetened natural peanut butter or almond butter

- ½ cup high quality cocoa powder

- Handful of coarse sea salt for garnishing

Instructions

- Preheat the oven to 350° F

- Mash or puree the bananas until smooth – should be about 1

½ cups of puree

- Put the bananas in a large bowl and add the peanut or almond butter and the cocoa powder

- Use a fork to mix together until the ingredients are fully combined in a smooth consistency

- Grease or line a cookie sheet and put spoonful's of the mixture onto the sheet, leaving about an inch between them

- Sprinkle a little sea salt over the top

- Bake for about 8-15 minutes until the sheen on the cookies has gone

- Remove from the oven and leave to cool for a few minutes before transferring them to a wire rack

Detox Pancakes Ingredients

- 1/3 cup rolled oats

- 2 tbsp. ground flax seeds

- ½ tsp baking powder – sodium free

- ½ tsp cinnamon

- 2 packed cups of raw spinach

- 3 large egg whites

- ½ bananas – medium ripe

- ½ tsp vanilla extract

Instructions

- Heat up a non-stick pan and coat it with cooking spray

- Blend the oats and flour together in a blender or food processor

- Empty into a bowl and then add the cinnamon, baking powder and flax seeds, stirring to combine thoroughly

- Put the spinach, banana, egg white and vanilla into a blender and pulse until smooth
- Add to the dry ingredients and stir until they are fully incorporated
- Spoon the batter into the hot pan and form four medium pancakes
- Cook for about 4-6 minutes on each side or until the edges have started to go brown
- Serve with fresh fruit, yogurt and nuts **Green Tea and Ginger Banana Ice Cream – Vegan Ingredients**
- 1 frozen banana – to freeze a banana, peel it and break it in half, freeze in a freezer-safe container until you need it
- ¼ cup of strong green tea, cold
- ½ cup non-dairy milk, unsweetened – almond or coconut milk are good for this
- ¼ inch knob of peeled ginger
- Pinch of sea salt
- Stevia to taste – no other sweetener as this is a pure natural one
- Almond slivers and chocolate chips or nibs

Instructions

- Blend the milk, banana, green tea, salt and ginger until very smooth and whipped – it should have the texture of soft-serve ice cream
- Add in stevia to taste if you want it
- Add the toppings and enjoy or blend the toppings in and freeze for about an hour before consuming

Raw Chocolate Mousse – Vegan Ingredients

- ½ cup of raw cashews, unsalted variety
- ½ cup of unsweetened coconut milk
- 10 drops of stevia liquid OR ½ tsp powdered stevia
- ¼ tsp vanilla extract
- 1 avocado, ripe
- 1 ½ tbsp. raw cacao powder
- Pinch of sea salt

Instructions

- Blend the cashews with the milk, vanilla extract and stevia liquid – if you used powder leave it out of this step
- When blended, add in the salt, cacao and avocado along with the powdered stevia if necessary.
- Adjust the taste for salt and sweetness
- Serve chilled, garnished with a sprinkling of cacao powder or cinnamon

Chocolate Coconut Pudding Ingredients

- 1 1/3 cup of unsweetened coconut milk
- 1 cup of raw cacao powder
- 1 cup of raw organic honey or natural maple syrup
- 1 cup of dates, chopped and pitted – measure after chopping
- ¾ cup of dark chocolate chips or nibs
- 1 ½ avocadoes
- 1 banana
- 3 tbsp. coconut oil. Melted
- 1 tsp vanilla extract

- Pinch of cinnamon

Instructions

- Blend all of the ingredients together in a blender except for the chocolate chips
- When blended, stir the chocolate chips in
- Pour into bowls or glass chars and refrigerate for several hours

Healthy Detox Cookies Ingredients

- 1 ½ cups of raw walnuts, halved
- 1 cup (about 12) pitted dates
- ¼ tsp salt
- ½ tsp baking soda
- 1 tsp vanilla extract
- 1 flax egg – mix 1 tbsp. of chia or flax seeds with 3 tablespoons water and refrigerate for 15 minutes before use
- ½ cup dark chocolate chips – optional

Instructions

- Preheat the oven to 350° F
- Line a cookie or baking sheet with a silpat or lining paper
- Use an "s" blade in the food processor to blend the walnuts and dates together – it should form a crumbly texture
- Add the vanilla, baking soda, salt and the flax egg to the mix and blend until it's all smooth and a bit stickier than traditional cookie dough is
- Add the chocolate chips and pulse quickly just to combine them
- Put spoonful's of batter onto the lined sheet and flatten them

gently with your hands – wet your hands a little first so the dough doesn't stick

- Bake for 12 minutes or until the edges have started turning golden

- Remove from the oven and leave to cool for 10 minutes before turning them out onto a wire rack

Gluten-free Strawberry Squares Ingredients

For the filling

- 2 tbsp. cornstarch

- 2 tbsp. warm water

- 2 cups of strawberries diced finely

- ¼ cup maple syrup or raw organic honey

- ¼ tsp stevia or truvia powder For the base and topping

- 2 ¼ cups quick oats – not the whole rolled variety

- 1 tsp ground cinnamon

- 1 cup almond butter, natural peanut butter or sunflower seed butter – unsalted

- ¼ cup maple syrup or raw organic honey

- ¼ cup of apple butter – do not use applesauce as it is not the same

- 1 large egg, beaten

- ½ cup almonds, sliced

Directions

- Make the filling by combining the cornstarch and the warm water until the cornstarch has completely dissolved – there should be no clumps and it should be the consistency of milk. Set to one side and mix the strawberries with the honey/syrup and stevia in a pan over a medium heat

- Bring the pan to a boil and stir it well
- Remove from the heat and stir the cornstarch in, whisking it until it is smooth. Leave to cool
- Preheat the oven to 325° F and line an 8 x 8 baking tray with foil, enough so that it hangs over the edges of the tray
- Make the base and topping by combining the oats, apple butter, honey/syrup, cinnamon, almond butter and egg together. Combine until the oats have been moistened and all the ingredients are thoroughly mixed together.
- Press half of the mixture onto the baking tray and press it down firmly and evenly.
- Spread the strawberry mixture evenly over the top
- Add the almonds to the rest of the oat mixture and then crumble it over the top of the strawberry mixture
- Use a wooden spoon or spatula to press it down into the filling firmly – it must stick well
- Bake for about 25-30 minutes until the top has browned lightly
- Cool completely before you cut into squares

Blueberry Almond Muffins Ingredients for 6 muffins

- 1 cup of rice flour, brown
- ½ tsp baking soda
- 1 tsp baking powder
- ¼ tsp salt
- 7-8 large dates, dried
- ½ cup of unsweetened soy or almond milk

- 1 ½ tbsp. coarse ground flax seeds

- 1 tbsp. lemon juice

- ½ tsp lemon zest

- 1/3 cup applesauce, unsweetened

- ½ tsp vanilla extract

- ½ cup fresh blueberries

- ¼ cup toasted sliced almonds

Instructions

- Preheat the oven to 400° F

- Put liners into a 6 cup muffin pan

- Pulse the dates in a blender until they are finely chopped

- Add the applesauce and blend until the mixture is a smooth paste

- Combine the vanilla extract, milk, lemon zest and juice together and add the ground flax seed. Mix well and set to one side

- Whisk the rice flour, baking powder, baking soda and salt together and then add the wet ingredients. Mix until they are just combined

- Add in the almonds and blueberries and stir gently

- Spoon the batter into the 6 cups and bake in the center of the oven for 20-25 minutes – test with a toothpick. When it comes out clean, they are cooked

- Remove and allow to cool for 10 minutes or so before turning them out onto a wire rack

Cherry Garcia Ice Cream – Vegan and Detox Ingredients

- 2 cans full fat coconut milk – 15 oz. each
- 3 droppers of vanilla flavored stevia
- Pinch of salt
- 2 ½ tbsp. cornstarch
- 1 cup cherries, roughly chopped – frozen is fine
- 3 or 4 cherries extra for the base
- ½ cup chopped dark chocolate

Instructions

- Put all ingredients except for the cornstarch, stevia, salt and ¼ cup of the coconut milk together in a pan
- Bring up to a simmer
- Whisk the cornstarch with the rest of the milk until smooth and add to the saucepan
- Cook, stirring well, until the mixture has thickened up and coats the back of a wooden spoon
- Remove the pan from the heat and leave to cool to room temperature
- Put the mixture into a blender and add the remaining cherries; blend until the base is smooth and a light pink color
- Cover, chill for at least 4 hours, up to 24 hours
- Freeze in an ice cream maker as per the manufacturer's instructions and in the last couple of minutes, add in the cherry and chocolate mix. Serve straight away or put into the freezer.

Chapter 5:

How to Detox Your Body Every Day

At the end of the day, we are all human beings. We all indulge at some time in our lives, admittedly some more than others and, in all honesty, there isn't any harm in the occasional glass of wine or a decadent dessert. It's when we do it all the time without taking preventative measures that the problems build up. There are things you can do every day that will help your body to detox, not just from the food you eat but from the daily onslaught of toxins, over which we have no control.

If you can't bear the thought of preparing for an intense detox, with a few changes to your diet and following the tips below, you can begin the process of detoxing your body every single day.

Drink Hot Lemon Water Every Morning

Drink a cup of hot or warm water with fresh lemon and cayenne every morning to kick-start your digestive system

Drink Cold Fresh-Pressed Juice

Preferably, on an empty stomach as your body will be able to better absorb all the nutrients. Try juicing kale, lemon, spinach, ginger and spirulina together!

Sip on a Detox Tea

Try a few cups throughout the day instead of water or coffee. Look for those that have licorice root, dandelion root, burdock and ginger in them

Use Apple Cider Vinegar

As often as you can, even add it to your juices and smoothies, or a teaspoon in your water. Apple cider vinegar alkalizes an acidic body and helps the liver to detox.

Eat Foods and Supplements That Detox

There are loads of different foods that you can choose from to help your liver and kidneys cleanse the body, including:

- Parsley
- Cilantro
- Dandelion root
- Licorice root
- Cayenne
- Turmeric
- Red pepper
- Garlic
- Lemon
- Lime
- Grapefruit
- Sea vegetables
- Beets
- Artichokes
- Cruciferous vegetables
- Spirulina
- Wheatgrass
- Chlorella
- Milk thistle

There are many more listed in this book that you can choose from as well

Eat Clean

More fiber in your diet to ensure your elimination process keeps on moving along smoothly. Limit the amount of fish that have a higher level of mercury such as:

- Swordfish
- Tuna
- Mackerel
- Shark
- Grouper
- Marlin

As a rule, the larger the fish, the more mercury it has. Avoid those processed foods, refined sugars, caffeine, alcohol and fruits or vegetables that are not organic.

Sweat it Out

As we discussed earlier, in order to get rid of toxins, you need to sweat. A sauna, light exercise, gardening, anything like that which makes you sweat will ultimately make your body cleaner and help to eliminate toxins. You can also try yoga.

Invert

Inverting has been categorically shown to stimulate the endocrine, lymphatic, nervous and cardiovascular systems because it reverses the flow of gravity. Some inversions you could have a go at are:

- A shoulder stand
- A headstand
- A hand stand
- Lying with your legs up against a wall

Jump

This is another activity that is good for stimulating circulation and the lymphatic system. Get a small portable trampoline and start adding jumping into your day.

Eliminate

Make sure you are getting plenty of fiber in your diet, as well as digestive enzymes, probiotics and go for a regular enema or colonic to keep your system clear.

Dry Body Brushing

Before you get in the shower or a bath, dry brush your entire body. Use lone strides of the brush towards the heart as this helps to get the lymphatic system activated and stimulates circulation, as well as helping to eliminate those toxins through the skin

Scrape Your Tongue

I bet you didn't expect to see that on the list! The tongue is the perfect place for bacteria to gather and any toxic debris that might have gathered overnight. Try and do this twice a day, while you are brushing your teeth and you will find that it helps enormously in releasing toxins from your body.

Hydrotherapy

Hydrotherapy sounds expensive and complicated but you can actually do this at home. Stand in your shower and turn the water on hot. After 30 seconds, turn it to cold and keep repeating this while you shower. The cold water helps to contract your blood vessels while the hot water causes them to dilate. By alternating hot and cold, your body's elimination process will be improved, inflammation decreases, waste is eliminated from body tissues and your circulation increased.

Detox Bath

This ideal to use after you have dry brushed your body. You should definitely have one of these baths one a week to help cleanse your system:

- 2 cups of Epsom salts
- 2 cups baking soda
- 1 tbsp. fresh ground ginger
- 4 drops each of geranium, juniper berry and eucalyptus essential oils

Add to your bath water and enjoy. Do make sure the essential oils are of the therapeutic grade, not the perfume grade as there is a vast difference between the two! The Epsom salts draw toxins out of the body through the skin, the baking soda alkalizes acid in the body and removes toxins while the ginger will heat up your temperature, helping you to perspire and we know that sweating is good for ridding us of toxins.

Make your House Healthy

Plants, like peace lilies, palms and ferns act as air filters, as well as looking nice. You should also make sure you change your air conditioning filters on a regular basis, do not use harsh household chemicals, have chlorine filters installed, get an air purifier and think about a reverse osmosis water system.

Detox Massage

One of the best forms of massage for inclusion in a detox plan is the manual lymphatic drainage massage. This form of massage uses gently strokes to stimulate the lymphatic system, encouraging it to eliminate any excess fluid, metabolic waste and bacteria. The effects of this kind of massage are many and includes benefits to the muscular system and the nervous system. It is a great addition to your detox plan as it encourages the fluid in the connective tissues to flow.

The lymphatic system is made up of lymph nodes, lymph vessels and organs. The lymph nodes are part of the defense system in the human body and they are responsible for removing microorganisms and other foreign bodies. They are a filter that keeps things like bacteria from getting into your blood stream and when the system becomes sluggish, all manner of things can get through.

Stimulating the lymphatic system through this kind of massage activates all of the system and it encourages cell regeneration and fluid circulation. Both of these are vital to proper detoxification, to speed up the healing process and to provide support to the immune system. Positive Health Online author, David Goddard ND, says:

"The lymphatic system has a vital role in the body by regulating the immune system, which protects the body against infection. It transports nutrients to cells and eliminates metabolic wastes, toxins and excess fluids from the body. Manual lymphatic drainage is also a very effective way of detoxing the body plus stimulating vital immune defenses. This is a powerful, deep cleansing treatment."

The Benefits of Manual Lymphatic Drainage

The real benefits of manual lymphatic drainage are:

- Clears congested areas, like puffy eyes, swollen ankles and swollen legs
- Promotes the healing of scar tissue, sprains, and torn ligaments
- Promotes post-operative healing
- Relieves swelling after plastic surgery
- Treats lymphedema and other conditions that may arise from venous insufficiency
- Promotes improvement in chronic conditions, like arthritis, sinusitis, acne and many other skin conditions

- Promotes deep relaxation

Do be careful to choose a properly trained therapist as this is a specific technique and must be done properly.

Simple Lymphatic Drainage – DIY

There is a way of helping your lymphatic system to drain and start moving again:

- Relax your fingers and place them gently on the sides of your neck, right underneath your ears
- Move the skin gently towards the back of your neck, using a downward motion
- Repeat this 10 times, moving your fingers gradually lower, away from your ears
- Now put your finger on either side of your neck at the tops of your shoulders
- Massage gently, moving the skin in towards the collarbone
- Repeat this 5 times.

Chapter 6:

7 Steps to Detox for Acne

It is so easy to forget that all of our body is connected and that the lifestyle you lead has an impact on all of the different parts. By giving your body a good detox, you are cleansing it of all impurities and allowing all of your organs to work together in perfect harmony, as they should do. Your skin is the largest organ you have and it too will benefit greatly from cleansing, to allow all the impurities to come out and be replaced with minerals and nutrients needed for healthy and clear skin. The following steps are designed to help you prevent acne from breaking out:

Step 1 – Stop the toxins from flooding in

Part of the process of detoxing your body is to significantly reduce the amount of toxins that are going into it. Toxins come in many disguises and some may not be quite as obvious as others. Alcohol and tobacco smoke are obviously toxic but how many of you realize just how many different pesticides and herbicides you are taking in from fruits and vegetables you eat that are grown conventionally? What about the meat and dairy products you eat – many of those are full of antibiotics and growth hormones. Add to that the heavy metals that are taken into your body over time and your body will soon become blocked. One of the side effects of all these toxins is acne.

Step 2 – Start from the inside

Acne comes from within your skin so it makes sense for you to target the problem or prevent it from happening from the inside out. Acne isn't an indicator of what you may be doing in your life now, rather it indicates things that you have or haven't done over the last few years. Move the focus of your treatment to the inside of your body and you will see improvements within a short period of time. Keep the treatment up and the long term effects will be even more obvious:

- Drink lots of water – at least 2 liter per day. Dehydration can make acne worse.

- Do a colon cleanse. When waste builds up in your colon, it can manifest itself in unhealthy skin. Make sure you avoid caffeine and alcohol and eat foods that target the live

- Eat plenty of organic vegetables and fruits, as well as grass-fed organic meats and dairy products to limit your toxic consumption

- If you smoke, stop.

- Shower in filtered water to limit how much chlorine gets on your skin

Step 3 – Only use natural treatments for acne

Instead of using chemical laden treatments that can be harsh on the skin, use products that are natural and organic. Not only will these reduce the side effects of the chemical ones, they will also provide your skin with nourishment in the form of plants and herbs. Give your body what it needs, not chemical substances but all natural things.

Step 4 – Use a healing detox facemask

If you suffer from a severe acne problem, try using a healing detox facemask that is made with bentonite clay. This is known for its properties that draw toxins from the skin and is often used as part of the detox bath treatment. It will clear out your pores, removing impurities and any ingrained dirt, and if you use it on a weekly basis, it will help to keep your skin clean and glowing.

Step 5 – Watch the results

Some people expect to see instant results during a detox but, more often than not, things will get worse before they get better. This is because your body is pushing all those impurities out and, if you have never done an acne detox before, you might be a little worried at the initial results. Establishing good habits and allowing plenty of time to pass will provide you with the real results – better looking healthy skin that is free of impurities.

Step 6 – Fill in the gaps in your nutrition

Speak to your nutritionist to see if they think your acne could be caused by deficiencies in nutrients. You may not be getting enough of certain mineral or vitamin from what you are eating and this could be causing the problem. You may need to take supplements so make sure you go for the whole food vitamins, as these do not contain any synthetic materials

Step 7 – Keep it up

Getting on top of your acne and staying on top is not a quick sprint, instead it is more like a marathon. Yes, you may

well want your acne to disappear in a flash but there is no miracle cure and your body needs time to adjust to all the changes you are making. Trying to speed thing sup will just make things worse so take it easy, take your time and you will see the results you want.

Chapter 7:

7 Steps to Making Your Own Detox Body Wrap

The detox body wrap is fast becoming one of the more popular detox methods and it involves wrapping your body to help the toxins to draw out. There are a few ways to do this so you should choose the type of wrap that suits your current situation. Completing all of these steps should afford you a nice feeling of wellbeing and you will be at the start of your journey for better health.

Step 1 – Decide which type of wrap you want

There are a number of different wraps, each one having a different goal. Some are designed to draw the toxins out from the skin and use bentonite clay. There are wraps that just remove the impurities from your skin by doing a deep cleanse on the outer lay. And there are wraps that help you to work up a sweat and are designed with weight loss in mind as well. You will need to use a sauna unit for these to work so that the exceed water weight can be sweated out while your body is being infused with herbs and minerals. Choose the one that suits your requirements before you move on to the next step

Step 2 – Get everything together

Now you know which type of wrap you are going for, you will need to get everything together. You do need to get your bathroom ready for what you are about to do so cover all the surfaces with plastic wrap to keep them clean. This is easy than using sheets or towels because you won't need to wash the plastic wrap, just discard it and it will cover better. It will also avoid any staining as some of the clays and lotions you will need to use can stain worktops and fabrics

You will need elastic bandages to wrap yourself up in, the solution you have chosen for your body wrap and a sauna unit if necessary. Have plenty of clean towels to hand and a few spare as well

Step 3 – Prepare your space

Make sure you have plenty of room and that you will be able to move around without banging into things once you are wrapped. Move wastebaskets out of the way and clear off the countertops. This is meant to be a relaxing experience so the last thing you want to do is keep tripping over things.

Step 4 - Prepare your wrap

Follow the instructions on the detox solution you are using. Most of them involve soaking the bandage in the solution and then wrapping them around yourself. Do follow any specific instructions to the letter so that you don't miss anything out. You will likely only have enough of the solution to do this once so there is no room for mistakes and you don't want to run out before you have finished covering yourself.

Step 5 – Wrap up

Before you start, have a shower to make sure you are clean. If you feel it necessary, exfoliate your skin as well this may make the detox solution soak in a little better. Start wrapping from your feet and work your way up your body, leaving your arms until last – you may need a little help to do the last one. If you are using the sauna nit method, get in; if not, lay in the bathtub – an empty one – so that the solution does not stain anywhere else. Cover the bathtub with plastic wrap first and make sure the room is a comfortable temperature.

Step 6 – Relax your body and mind

It might seem hard to relax while you are wrapped up like a mummy but if you start with your mind, your body will follow. Think positive thoughts. Detoxing isn't just about the body; it is also about the mind and ridding it of toxic thoughts. Think of things that make you feel good or think about what you are doing and the results you are hoping to achieve.

Step 7 – Unwrap

Once the set time has passed, normally at least an hour, you can start to unwrap your body. This is usually done in the reverse order. Unclasp the wraps and allow them to unravel. When you are unwrapped, take a cool shower to rinse off the solution and impurities and then dry off.

How Detox Wraps Work

The detox solution that you are using will be full of clay, minerals r specific herbs that are desired to draw toxins out of your body. While you can use these solutions on their own, using a wrap adds pressure, which increases the chances of absorption. The detox wrap is an active way of getting the toxins to come out of your body, as opposed to the detox bath, which is a passive way.

Chapter 8:

5 Homemade Detox Hair Masks and Shampoos

The hair care industry is raking in billions of dollars every single year but you don't need to contribute to that if you really don't want to. You can easily make your own detox shampoo and hair masks to help remove the toxins and the chemical buildup from your scalp. The following recipes are easy to make and the results will be tremendous.

Shampoos

Use these to cleanse your scalp and effectively get rid of the chemical build up and impurities that are left behind by traditional shampoos and hair care products.

Lemon and Cucumber

The lemon will clean your scalp a treat and the cucumber works to cool and calm things down a little. This is a dead easy recipe to make and is ideal for those who have a dry and itchy scalp.

Ingredients

- 1 fresh lemon, peeled
- 1 fresh cucumber, peeled
- Olive oil – optional
- Rosemary essential oil – optional

Instructions

- Blend the lemon and cucumber in your blender
- Massage into your hair and leave for a few minutes, then rinse out thoroughly

You can add olive oil or rosemary oil blended with the lemon first and then sieved through before blending with the cucumber. If you hair is dry, use more cucumber and if your hair is oily, use more lemon.

Natural pH Balanced Shampoo

If you think the pH levels of your hair are wrong, this shampoo is a great way to put everything back in balance. The recipe is simple to follow and you get all the natural goodness from the ingredients straight to your scalp and hair. The beauty of this recipe is that you can make a large batch and preserve it until you need it.

Ingredients

- 1 can of coconut milk. If you prefer making your own, use about 1 ½ cups
- 1 ¾ cups aloe Vera gel
- Essential oils – optional

Instructions

- Mix the ingredients together with a wire whisk until fully combined
- Pour the mixture out into ice cube trays
- Freeze for a few hours until completely frozen.
- Take one cube out and defrost it thoroughly in a bowl
- Wet your hair and then massage the shampoo into your scalp and gradually work it towards the ends of your hair
- Leave it for 30 seconds or so and then rinse

Do not keep adding more because you cannot see any lather – this recipe does not lather and a little works wonders. You can rinse your hair off using apple cider vinegar as well because this will ensure that all traces are removed. If your ice cubes are large, only use a quarter or half and sore the rest in the refrigerator for up to one week

Coconut Milk Shampoo

Using coconut in your shampoo gives your hair a real treat – plenty of nutrients and fats that will help it to grow. This recipe can also be used as a body wash in the shower.

Ingredients

- 1/3 cup of coconut milk – homemade is best
- ½ cup coconut oil soap
- 2 tsp sweet almond oil
- 10 drops lavender essential oil - optional

Instructions

- Place all the ingredients in a jar and shake well to combine
- Pour out into a squeeze bottle and use as needed
- Shake well before use

Hair Masks

These masks will penetrate deeply into your hair, providing nutrition and an immediate change in the texture and health of your hair.

Aloe and Clay Detox Mask

This recipe calls for bentonite clay and aloe Vera gel to help moisturize your hair. The recipe is easy to follow and inexpensive.

Ingredients

- ½ cup bentonite clay powder
- ½ cup aloe Vera gel

- ¼ cup apple cider vinegar
- 1 extra cup of apple cider vinegar

Instructions

- Mix the clay powder, allow Vera gel and the ¼ cup of apple cider vinegar together until thoroughly combined
- Work it into your hair, massaging it in
- Put a shower cap on and leave it for about 20-30 minutes – do NOT allow it to dry onto your hair
- Rinse it off with 1 cup of apple cider vinegar and leave it for between 1 and 3 minutes before shampooing.

Natural Clay Mud Mask

This is a very simple but highly effective mud mask that can be made with Redmond or bentonite clay> the latter is usually used for detoxing because it has a very powerful drawing effect, pulling toxins out and leaving the hair feeling fresh and new. Essential oils are recommended but be aware that some herbs can darken or lighten your hair. Nettle leaf can be used on any color or type of hair; chamomile flowers are best for light colored hair while rosemary oil is good for dark hair.

For dark hair, mix ¼ cup of rosemary leaf with 2 tbsp. nettle leaf and 2 cups of boiling water. For blonde hair, use 2 tbsp. of nettle leaf and ¼ cup of chamomile flowers in 2 cups of boiling water. Cool and strain into 2 cups

Ingredients

- Herbal tea as per above suggestions
- ½ cup apple cider vinegar
- ¾ cup of Redmond or bentonite clay
- 10 drops of your favorite essential oil – tip – rosemary and lavender oils promote hair growth

Instructions

- Brew the tea and leave it to cool

- Strain thoroughly into t 2 cups

- Pour one cup into the blender and add the apple cider vinegar. If the blades are metal, pour the mixture

into a plastic bowl instead

- Add the clay a bit at a time, mixing well with a non-metal spoon or whisk to incorporate it thoroughly

– the eventual consistency should be like yoghurt

- Add the essential oils and mix them in thoroughly

- Wet your hair and massage a handful of the mixture in,

stating from the roots and going all the way to end of the hair – use as much mixture as needed

- Leave it for between 5 and 20 minutes but do not let it dry

- Rinse with 1 cup of herbal tea mixed with a tbsp. of apple cider vinegar

Chapter 9:

Essential Oils for Body and Mind Detox

Essential oils have been proven time and again to have properties that serve our health, our physical wellbeing and our emotional wellbeing. However, some of them can also act as very powerful detoxification aids for both the body and the mind. These oils can be used alone or mixed as a combination. They must be diluted and can be applied topically on the skin, added to your bah or inhaled. You can also use a diffuse in some cases.

When you use essential oils in your bath water, you must wait until the bath is as full as you want it before you sprinkle in the old – anywhere from 8 to 30 drops, depending on how strong you want it to be. This is because the oils evaporate very quickly and you won't get the full benefit if you add them while the water is running. Do not immerse yourself under the water, as essential oils are irritating to the eyes. Also, if you are using them in the bath, do not use any other soap as some can neutralize the oils and interfere with the way they work.

Some of the best oils, known to have detoxification properties are

- Rose
- Black pepper
- Cypress
- Juniper berry
- Fennel

- Coriander

- Sage

- Parsley

- Frankincense

- Carrot seed

- Grapefruit

- Bitter orange

- Lemon

- Nutmeg

- Peppermint

- Laurel

- Rosemary

- Mandarin

- Hyssop

- Patchouli

- Helichrysum

Always blend your chosen oils in a carrier oil like olive oil, vegetable oil or almond oil before you used them in the bath or on your skin

10 Essential Oils That Will Detox and Purify Your Body

The true beauty of these oils comes in the fact that they have so many different uses, depending on what you need them for. Detoxing is the act of helping to rid the body of all the toxic waste, the negative thoughts you may be having, anxiety, stress and any harmful organisms in the body and these oils contain many benefits.

1. Peppermint Oil

Peppermint oil can be used in a number of ways. First, you can add a few drops to your bath water. Second, you can use it topically; you can add water to a few drops of it and drink it or you can pop a few drops in your detox smoothie or tea.

Peppermint oil is good for helping you to get your concentration levels back up and to maintain them, as well as being soothing for the digestive system. It comes from the peppermint plant, which has been used for medicinal use for thousands of years. It is often mixed with other oils for a true detoxifying blend.

2. Juniper Oil

Juniper oil is derived from the juniper berry, which are also great for the body because of all the antioxidants they contain. They are a great aid for your digestive system and as a diuretic. Using the oil means that you are getting the full essence of the plant without having to use the actual plant.

Juniper oil is good for detoxifying and soothing the mind, to help you alleviate stress and pain. Used as a diuretic, it can flush out toxins and help to get rid of a buildup in water weight, which includes excess sodium.

3. Grapefruit Oil

You may be used to eating grapefruit or drinking grapefruit juice but you may not have known that the oil extracted from the fruit can be of huge help to the body in many ways. One of its properties is that it can help to detoxify the body and it could be the most useful of all the essential oils. Not only that, it does not have to be used just as part of a detox program; grapefruit oil can be used daily to keep your body healthy.

Grapefruit oil has also been scientifically shown to kill off viruses that may be roaming your body, as well as any troublesome microbes. Lastly, it is used as a diuretic, helping to flush toxins and waste out of your body.

4. Rosemary Oil

Maybe you use rosemary as an herb in the kitchen and maybe you just grow it because of its wonderful smell. The oil that comes from the rosemary plant is highly detoxifying, as well as being good for the whole body. If you take the healthy properties of the rosemary plant and put them in an oil, you get the benefits, such an improvement to your digestive system, better circulation, diuretic properties and anti-inflammatory properties.

Rosemary has been shown to fight off memory loss and cancer. It can be inhaled in aromatherapy or you can use it in your bath. You can even add it to massage oil and use it during a massage.

5. Laurel Oil

Laurel oil is derived from the laurel leaf and these have been shown to contain vast amounts of healthy antioxidants that can give your body a boost in more ways than one. Instead of attempting to consume the actual leaf, you get the same benefits from the oil. We all know that one of the top reasons for doing a detox is to get the digestive system moving again and laurel oil does just that; you only need a small amount of it as well. You can also add it to a diffuser to get into your body through the respiratory system.

6. Mandarin Oil

Mandarin oil comes from the fruit and has been shown to have amazing properties in helping to relax and soothe the nervous system. This is one of the best things you can do to get your body back on track and get it prepared to be detoxified. Mandarin oil also helps to purify the blood and can make improvements to your circulatory system.

Because it is derived from the fruit, it has a wonderful aroma and is a nice oil to use in aromatherapy. It helps to boost the function of the liver, which is the single most important organ in your body when it comes to detoxification. If your liver is not performing properly, neither will any of your other organs.

7. **Lemon Oil**

It has long been known that the lemon has highly astringent properties and is ideal to be used as part of a detoxification plan. Lemon oil is often added to the products you buy for cleaning because it smells nice and promotes a feeling of cleanliness. Some of the benefits of using lemon oil include cancer prevention properties, freeing up the respiratory system and helping the lymphatic system to function correctly. It can also be used as an anti-inflammatory. Lemon oil can be used in a bath, or added to a detox smoothie.

8. **Patchouli Oil**

Patchouli oil is derived from the plant of the same name and it has been shown to improve, not just your mind but your sex drive as well. Patchouli oil is an essential oil that doesn't get much press but it has some great benefits. It can be used in a detox plan for the body and the mind by adding a few drops to a warm bath. If you want to take advantage of the diuretic properties of patchouli oi, add a few drops to a glass of water, your detox smoothie, soup or tea.

9. **Hyssop Oil**

Hyssop oil is another one that isn't quite so well-known but, as its benefits become more widely known, it will get more popular. Hyssop oil is used as way of treating problems with the digestive system and that is where you need to start when you detox your body. The digestive system is the part of your body that is responsible for eliminating the most amount of toxins and if it stops working properly, it leaves your body at risk of other conditions and diseases.

10. Helichrysum Oil

You would be forgiven for wondering just how you were going to get more of this highly beneficial plant into your body on a daily basis and that is where helichrysum oil comes into play. Helichrysum is part of the sunflower family and it is chock full of benefits. Many of these target the skin and, as this is the largest organ of the body, it is one of the best for removing toxins. Helichrysum oil is useful for reducing the amount of inflammation in your body and in helping to regenerate cells.

Detox Blends

Not all oils will work the way you want them to and it isn't always easy to find the right blends. This section is designed to give you a few ideas of which oils to blend to help in your detox plan.

One of the most powerful blends of essential oils that is thought to have highly detoxifying effects on all of the organs in your boy, and your skin, is a mix of seaweed oil, juniper berry oil, fennel oil and lemon oil.

Another highly potent mix is fir oil, hyssop oil, fennel oil, patchouli oil and helichrysum oil, blended together with a base oil that is neutral. Live toxicity is often evidenced by pain in the lower and middle back and you may also get bad headaches. This blend of oils is cleansing and should be applied topically to the areas that are toxic. If you are not entirely sure which areas they are, apply it to areas of weakness or use it as an oil for massaging your feet.

A good blend for the lymphatic system and the liver is rosemary oil, geranium oil, roman chamomile oil, carrot seed oil, German chamomile oil, blue tansy oil and helichrysum oil. This potent blend works to cleanse the lymphatic system and the liver removing higher levels of toxins. It can also break up any angry areas in the liver. It should be applied topically, directly over the liver, the solar plexus or used as a full body massage oil.

For stress relief and a mind detox, use a blend of geranium oil, lavender oil, ylang ylang oil, sandalwood oil and blue tansy oil. This special blend helps to free your body of emotional trauma and is also a great blend for a liver detox and in times of distress. Apply topically over the solar plexus, liver and the forehead or use in a foot massage.

Please seek medical advice before you use any of these blends, especially if you are pregnant or are planning to fall pregnant.

Two Feel-Good Essential Oil Recipes

Anti-aging - blend 15 drops of ylang ylang oil with 5 drops of geranium oil into 50 ml of a vegetable oil. Massage it into the neck and face before going to sleep. You can also massage this into your scalp once a week, about 15 minutes before you shampoo your hair.

Anti-stress - this is a blend for a bath. Use 100 ml of a neutral base oil and add 50 drops of lavender oil, 50 drops of mandarin oil and 50 drops if ylang ylang oil. Add to the bath. If you want a tonifying oil, add in 60 drops of lemon oil and 50 drops of rosemary oil.

Bonus Chapters

How to Detox from Alcohol

People who only have the occasional drink will not need to worry about this but for the heavier drinker and those who are diagnosed alcoholics, I hope that this chapter will help you to understand and learn how you can help yourself by undergoing a home detox. Many people don't understand the seriousness of an alcohol detox, or understand how difficult it can be or the dangers of withdrawal.

There are two stages to an alcohol detox; the first starts 6-24 hours after the last drink and can last for up to 7 days. This is the most dangerous period of withdrawal and the person may need medical help. At the very least, they should be properly monitored, especially if this is being done at home, rather than in a detox center. The second stage is the longest and it takes place over a course of months as the brain starts to resume its normal function. It is in this stage when the sleep patterns start to return to normal and emotions come under control.

Preparation for Alcohol Detox at Home

Your Environment

One of the main reasons for wanting to do this in your own home, rather than at a detox center, is for the comfort factor. That's OK but there are certain rules that you must follow. First, you must understand that an alcohol detox and withdrawal does not take all that long but you won't be going anywhere while it's happening. You will have to stay home so make sure you have plenty of books and movies, games to play, whatever it takes to keep your mind off the alcohol. The next rule is, rid your house of all alcohol. There won't be any saving a bit for a special occasion, or keeping it just in case, it all has to go. Once those withdrawal symptoms kick in, you will be heading straight for your emergency stash.

Have a family member of a friend come and stay with you – you are going to need the support from the very first day. They need to be there for at least a few days but manly while you are going through the withdrawal symptoms.

Home remedies for alcohol detox

Dietary Changes

During alcohol detox, there will be times where you won't want to eat or won't be able to keep your food down. However, at this point in time, your diet is absolutely critical. You need to have the right foods and drinks on hand to help you. The idea behind this is the same as someone who is doing a detox diet except it is much more important. You need a house full of fresh fruits and vegetables, whether you like them or not.

This isn't about eating what you like because, if you fill up on moon pies or Cheetos, you are just swapping one problem for another. Instead, the fruits and vegetables are to help speed up the release of the toxins that are rushing around your body. Berries are a good choice have they are full of natural sugars and sugar is something that ex- drinkers want. Oats help to control your blood sugar and help to relax you. Bananas are good sources of energy as well as helping to boost your mood and are full of fiber and potassium. You want foods that are protein rich, like fish, chicken or peanut butter. You don't have to eat huge meals; eat little and often instead.

Don't eat junk or processed food; if you want the best results out of your detox, eat plenty of nutrient rich food. Junk food is full of refined sugar and bad carbohydrate, all increasing the toxins in the body. The idea of the detox is to get rid of these, not add more to them. You may not think that an apple will help you feel better but, trust me, it will in the long run.

Drink enough water

Water is vital to every person, not just those on a detox. You must drink large quantities of water every day but no more than 2 quarts an hour. You can throw a few fresh fruit juices in for a change but, primarily, your fluid intake has to come from water. Your withdrawal symptoms will ease and the toxins will be flushed out of your body that much quicker. Avoid drinking tea or coffee or any other drink that contains caffeine. Your sleep is already going to be disturbed and caffeine will just make that worse. In terms of water, you should be looking at around 100 ounces a day. This will wash the toxins and the chemicals right out of your body, as well as the alcohol and it will also help with the dehydration issues that surround alcohol consumption.

Have enough vitamin B

When you drink alcohol on a daily basis, your levels of vitamin B diminish, causing a deficiency. To help heal your body from the inside, you must make sure you replace that vitamin B as well as taking in sufficient to keep your levels up. You also need to restore vitamin C and magnesium to ensure that your body functions as smoothly as possible.

Use Milk Thistle & Kudzu

Milk thistle extract is a natural way of removing toxins from your body by stopping the liver from absorbing the alcohol and helping to reduce how severe the side effects are. Kudzu has been in use almost since time began as a form of treatment for alcohol consumption. It has powerful antioxidant properties that help to reduce the damage done to the liver and to help it regenerates. 10 grams of kudu powder daily is sufficient to curb the cravings for alcohol.

Use Angelica Extract

Angelica helps to reduce alcohol cravings and the withdrawal symptoms. It's an herb with anti-inflammatory properties that have the power to curb your desire to drink. 5 drops per day is the recommended dosage, added water. It will also help to reduce bloating and headaches that are commonly associated with alcohol abstinence.

Add Cayenne Pepper to Food

Cayenne pepper is another one that helps to curb the cravings and it will increase your appetite as well. Add it food to reduce symptoms of nausea and decreased appetite that come with a withdrawal from alcohol.

Drink Passion Flower Tea

Passion flower tea helps to alleviate interrupted sleep and symptoms of delirium, by relaxing your body and mind. Drink it as often as you want.

Basil

Basil is an extremely potent herb and one of the most effective at reducing cravings. It has both antioxidant and anti- inflammatory properties that help to eliminate free radicals and fully detoxify your body. The best way to take it is to soak fresh basil twigs in water overnight with 20 peppercorns.

Bitter Gourd Leaves

Bitter gourd leaves have been shown to help repair damaged livers. They are packed full of compounds that can help to cure alcoholism through flushing toxins out of the body. The leaves must be ground up to extract the juice and drink fresh in a glass of buttermilk.

Ashwagandha

Ashwagandha is one of those ancient herbs that are full of medicinal properties. It has both anti-oxidant and anti- inflammatory properties that help to detox the body while improving brain function at the same time. It can help to alleviate tension, stress and help you to feel better overall. Take one teaspoon with a glass of milk two time a day.

Gotu Kola

This is a supplement that helps to improve the functions of the brain and the nervous system. It also acts as a blood purifier, keep stress at bay and reduce anxiety. 50 grams should be taken three times a day.

All of these home remedies help to keep your stamina up so that you can better fight off the addiction and beat the withdrawal symptoms. As you can see from the list, most of these are included the detox diets we talked about earlier and can all help to rush the toxins out of the body much quicker than they would come out otherwise. The quicker the toxins leave, the quicker you will begin to feel better. Make no mistake though; the path to alcohol recovery is much longer than detoxing your body for a week but with the right help and support, this is one battle that you can win.

Dealing with Cravings

It is normal to experience cravings, they are part and parcel of any addiction and you will be keenly aware of them throughout withdrawal. They can also appear many weeks or months, even years in some cases, after you have kicked the habit. The following are some important facts about cravings that you need to know to learn how to deal with them:

What You Should Know About Cravings:

Cravings are not caused through a lack of motivation or willpower. They also do not mean that your withdrawal and detox is not working. Cravings actually last for a very short period of time and they are never there 24/7. What triggers cravings is some kind of emotional or physical upset or discomfort and managing that will help you to manage your cravings.

Things You Can Do to Manage Cravings:

You need to know what triggers a craving. It could be a person, a place, or something that reminds you of alcohol. Once you learn to identify the triggers, you need to learn to direct your mental energy elsewhere, to ways that will help you to avoid those triggers again.

Tell yourself constantly why you have stopped drinking and list down the negative effects of the alcohol on your life. List the positives to giving it up and staying clean as well.

Call on your support network for help when you need it.

Make sure you follow the home remedies for an alcohol detox. Detoxing your body will help these cravings to disappear quicker.

After the Alcohol Detox

About 36 hours into your detox, you will begin to feel very uncomfortable and irritable; this will last for up to a week. Do not, under any circumstances, stop your detox. In fact, at this stage, it is more important than ever that your diet is right and that you are maintaining your health and your detox routine. Make sure you are taking any vitamins and supplements that you need, getting a little exercise and sleeping.

It won't take long before you are able to get back to normal as long as you are not placed under any stress. What you have to understand here is that you have detoxed from the alcohol. The toxins are gone but, if you don't make significant changes to your lifestyle, you will soon be back where you started.

Once the alcohol is gone from your system, you will find that your appetite increases. This is where you should follow the detox guidelines up above to ensure that your body stays healthy and fit enough for you to fight off any cravings. You will also probably be very malnourished and will need to eat good whole foods to get your strength back up. Again, as I said before, eat small and often rather than trying to struggle though a big meal. Just make sure you are eating the right foods.

If this is the very first time you have had to go through an alcohol detox, be glad it is over. Learn from it and never put yourself back in the situation where you have to do it again. The principles of an alcohol detox are no different from any other detox; it is just a much harder experience to go through.

Don't Forget Your Pets

When we talk about detoxing, we always talk in terms of humans and we tend to forget about our pets. We all have a pretty good idea what toxins are and we also have an understanding of how they affect our health. We know that they can worsen any existing health problems but do you know how much the toxins that affect you affect your pets? The problem with toxins is that they are hidden and we are unwittingly causing both our animals and ourselves health problems that are not necessary. We already know how bad toxins are for us but, for your pets, they can be devastating, for a number of reasons.

First, your pets are smaller than you are and they have much smaller livers, kidneys and lungs, all the organs that help to eliminate the toxins. When they are exposed to toxins, those organs have to work so much harder to remove them. Second, they don't live as long as we do. They don't have the time for their bodies to eliminate those toxins on a gradual basis. They can't talk to us, tell us that something they are eating or breathing in is making them ill. They can't change their own food or stop using a cleaning fluid or spray that is irritating their lungs. They rely on us, their owners, 100% because we control the environment they live in and the food they eat.

So, how do you minimize the toxins that your pet is exposed to and help them to get rid of the ones they already have in their bodies? Before we look at how you can help them, let's take a deeper look at these toxins and how our cats and dogs come into contact with them.

Tracking the Toxins

There are several ways that your pet can be exposed to toxins. Some are through accidental ingestion. Weed killers, exhaust fumes, pesticides, motor oil, and chemical deicers get into our pets when they walk on grass, paths or roads, when they at grass coated in chemicals and lick dust and dirt off their coats and their paws. The air fresheners, household cleaners, washing products and any other chemical that we use in the household can also find their way into your pet's body. Toxins in the water, in commercially prepared dog foods and treats and in medications and shampoos we use on them. Some toxins are actually produced in their bodies, like ammonia, through their own metabolic processes or through bacteria or yeast in the GI tract.

In the wild, animals have a more efficient elimination system for flushing out toxins. These systems have developed over the years to counteract natural toxins in the environments they frequent but domesticated pets don't have the ability to combat the constant bombardment of toxins that they are faced with on a daily basis, mainly because their bodies have not had the years they need in which to adapt enough to fight the battle.

What Are The Ill Effects of Toxins?

When a body is healthy, the toxins are quickly eliminated through the lungs, kidneys and liver, as well as the intestines and the skin. Because domesticated pets have not adapted their elimination systems to cope with the sheer numbers of toxins, they react in pretty much the same way as we do – their bodies become inflamed, and they up their production of mucus or diarrhea to try to help the immune system to get rid of them.

When a body takes in too many toxins, it has to store the excess until there is a good time to get rid of them. For many pets, that good time will never come and the toxins simply continue to build up. Over time, you might notice that your dog or cat is lethargic, fatigues and prone to infections. The overload of toxins will eventually stop the immune system from working to the extent where they begin to suffer with tumors and cysts and, as the cells degrade even further, even more serious health problems will begin to manifest themselves.

There is good news though, most animals are perfectly well equipped to fight infection and disease, eliminate some toxins and to restore their internal organs and systems back to health but they do need your help. If you feed your pet a natural diet, with plenty of exercise and rest and playtime thrown in for good measure your pet will have a level of health that you would never have thought possible. In short, you can give them a new lease of life by following the 15 steps below to detoxing your pet.

Fifteen Steps to Detox Your Pet

Give them better quality food and treats

This is always your first port of call in proving the life and longevity of your pet. If you feed your pet on cheap supermarket brand foods, you are feeding them chemicals, in the form of additives, artificial flavoring and coloring. Commercial foods also contain low quality fillers and proteins that are hard on your pet's digestive system, as well as increasing the toxins in the body. Instead, go for high quality natural foods and treats. It may be more expensive but you cannot put a price on your pet's life.

Only Filtered Water

While your tap water may be classed as fit to drink, it is full of toxins, in the form of certain minerals and metals, along with the chemicals that are added to keep it clean – chlorine and fluoride for starters. There are even going to be trace amounts of compounds that are similar to hormones and a number of other suspicious things that will harm the health of your pet. Water filtration units are not expensive and you can buy them almost anywhere.

Add Herbs and Nutrient Supplements

There are lots of herbs and natural supplements that you can add to your pet's food that will help cleanse their systems. Lots of these nutrients are usually missing from commercially prepared foods, such as amino acids, antioxidants, chlorophyll, essential fatty acids and trace minerals. Do your homework and find good quality supplements with cleansing herbs that will help your dog to live a longer and healthier life.

Cut out Household Chemicals

As well as the obvious ones, such as fly sprays, cleaning chemicals and solvents, there are also toxins fond in perfumes, deodorants, air fresheners, plug in air fresheners, washing products and tumble dryer sheets. These tend to be full of chemicals that are not regulated and are not tested by health protection agencies and many of them have been prove to have an adverse effect on breathing problems in both people and pets. Either use only 100% natural products or make your own. Ingredients like lemon, vinegar, and baking soda all make excellent cleaning products and they are all natural and non-toxic.

Exercise Every Day

You need to get your body moving to help eliminate toxins and so does your pet. Exercise speeds up the elimination process by moving waste products through the digestive tract. It also improves blood and lymph fluid circulation, which are the two main means your pet uses for moving debris and toxins through the body. Exercises also help to improve respiration, which allows the excess toxins to be removed from the respiratory tract. If you can't get out for a walk with them every day, make sure you give them exercise in other ways by playing with them in the garden – and that includes the cat!

Improve the Quality of the Air

Pollution can come from all directions and indoors it comes from household cleaner chemicals, perfumes, deodorants, air fresheners and cigarette or cigar smoke. It can also come from synthetic furnishings like carpets, cushion covers or flooring, even the furniture itself. If your new furniture is giving off the aroma of "new", make sure you keep your pets away from the areal and keep windows open to ventilate the area well. You can also use window fans and bathroom fans to remove the effects of hairspray and perfume, or other things that you regularly spray around.

Minimize the Amount of Outdoor Chemicals they are Exposed to

If your pets spend time outside, they will come into contact with a number of different chemicals – pest control, fertilizers, weed killers and much more. If your dog eats grass, watch them while you are out walking, especially in public places where chemicals are likely to have been used. You can eliminate this behavior by adding in greens to their food, both cats and dogs. You can actually grow cat grass, which is free of the toxic contaminants.

Reduce the Amount of Conventional Medications You Use

There are a lot of toxic chemicals and compounds in traditional treatments for fleas and ticks, not to mention worm tablets and vaccines, as well as lots of other drugs that your pet may need. While these treatments may be a necessary part of owning a pet, you can keep in check how much they are exposed to. Don't over dose them on the flea and tick treatments, only administer medications when it is absolutely necessary and, where you can look for alternative treatments. For example, using lemons, rosemary and water and spraying it once a week can make a good flea and tick treatment. It's also much cheaper than having to use what your veterinary practitioner sells. Think about the vaccines your dog has every year – it doesn't actually need them and it has been proven that they are not necessary and can be dangerous to the health of your pet, as well as decreasing their lifespan naturally.

Support their Liver

The liver is the main vehicle used for eliminating toxins, not just in humans but in animals too. Make sure your pet has the right antioxidants in his or her diet as these help the liver to work more efficiently. Use herbs like milk thistle, added to their food every day, to boost the liver function. While your pet is young and healthy, it probably won't need any liver support but older animals and those that are on medications will do. Please make sure you speak with a holistic vet before giving your dog or cat anything as he or she is trained to advise you what you should, or shouldn't as the case may be, using.

Provide Support for the Immune System

In the same way that yours does, your pet's immune system works with their organs to keep them well. To support their immune system, you are helping to keep their lungs, liver, kidneys and intestines healthy as well as their skin so that their natural detoxification system will work properly. If you want your pets to be healthy, feed them a high quality mineral and multivitamin supplement, one that is designed for pets, not humans. For older pets or those that are very active, you can also give them pet antioxidant supplements.

Help their Skin to Breathe

Cats and dogs use their skin to eliminate toxins and regular brushing helps it to breathe, which allows the toxins to come out. It also gets rid of any dust and rubbish that may accumulated on their coats, debris that could contain chemical residues, thus making sure your reduce the amount of toxins ingested when they groom themselves. For dogs, look at the bathing products you are using. Are they high quality, made from natural products? Always use natural grooming products to cut down on the amount of toxins your pet take in when you are bathing him or her.

Don't forget, although they remove toxins through their skin, it is also a way in.

Support Their Digestive System

When your pet digests toxins, many of them are eliminated through the colon and keeping their digestive system healthy means that the toxins move n before they get the chance to do any damage to the walls of the intestines or are reabsorbed back into the body. If your pet has a sluggish or irritated bowel, he or she may have chronic diarrhea and this suggests that something is not right inside. If your pet is constipated, the toxins can go back into their blood before they can be eliminated, further complicating the problem. Bacteria and yeast are capable of producing toxins, which can have an adverse effect so make sure you give your pet probiotics, enzymes or a complete supplement that is designed to support the gastrointestinal system.

Support Their Kidneys

The easiest and simplest thing to do to help support your pet's kidneys in make sure they are drinking sufficient amounts of filtered water daily. Toxins that are eliminated through the kidneys can be highly concentrated if your pet is dehydrated and this can damage the structures that make up the filtration system in the kidneys. Also, mineral particles form if the urine is concentrated, which could result in crystals or stones form that can block up or irritate the urinary tract. This can be the start of numerous infections that simply won't go away or keep coming back. If your dog or cat is not a big drinker, add water or broth into their food. Cats in particular will drink very little so keep them on a high quality wet diet where possible. If you feed them on the pouches or cans of food, add a little warm water to the pouch or can afterwards and add it to the food. Not only does this increase their hydration, it also ensures that they are getting all of the goodness out of the food because none of the jelly or gravy is left behind.

Keep Things Clean

The home environment has been shown to have far worse air quality than outdoors. However, a certain mount of the toxins in our houses comes in from outdoors as dust or other pollutants. Dust, vacuum and clean regularly to keep these toxins down and reduce the amount of toxic matter that your pet can ingest. Also, be very strict about cleaning their beds on a regular basis and their food and water bowls.

Use Herbs and Homeopathic Remedies to Help Your Pet Detox

Because they live with us and because we are responsible for their wellbeing, it is up to us to keep the levels of the toxins down. However, all pets can benefit from regular and gentle detoxing, which you can do with the aid of herbs and other homeopathic remedies that can help to support their organs, cleanse their systems and help them to eliminate toxins better. Again, please seek advice from a registered holistic vet before you give your pet any supplements.

Rules of the Detox Diet

As you probably know by now, there are several different meanings to the word "detox", all of which differ based on the affect they have on your body. One of the most popular goals of a detox program is to purify the body and cleanse it of all of the unclean toxins that it has become infested by during our normal routines.

This buildup of toxicity in your body is obviously something to be alarmed about. After all, any foreign toxic chemical simply being present in your body in trace amounts is enough to send anybody to the doctor, or at least make a major shift in their lifestyle choices in order to facilitate a healthier body. However, although serious, the buildup of toxic chemicals that detoxification is supposed to reverse should not come as a surprise to you given the way we live our lives in today's modern day and age, an age where once widely accepted traditions of health are now ignored for the sake of convenience.

In our normal every day routines what do we eat? Processed sugars, preservatives, corn syrup, saturated fats, such chemicals that we would be averse to should we see them in their true form are eaten in large quantities because they make the food we eat and the beverages we drink taste better. Eating fast food has become a regular, every day portion of our lives, we actually eat these poisonous foods for fun! Even when we eat at home, we often accompany our drinks with carbonated beverages or alcohol.

When not consuming alcohol with meals, we often consume it for enjoyment whilst socializing. Getting heavily inebriated due to the consumption of alcohol has become an extremely common past time for the average person in today's modern day and age.

Additionally, we fuel our increasingly work oriented and fast paced lives through the use of stimulants such as caffeine and nicotine, the latter of which often brings with it substances as toxic as tar and cyanide due to the method via which it is most commonly consumed. Caffeine providing beverages and foods are not all that much better, for they obstruct your body's natural system as well.

With all of these unimaginably toxic substances being pumped by us into our very own bodies, willingly at that, it should not come as a surprise that these toxins build up in our bodies and prevent it from functioning the way it should.

The best way to fix this problem is via a detox diet which not only cuts you off from all of these poisonous chemicals, it also makes you eat the kinds of foods that allow your body to cleanse itself and clean out all of the toxins from within it more efficiently.

Here is a list of some of the rules you will need to be following while you are on your detox diet:

>Complete avoidance of all stimulants and depressants: This one should be pretty obvious but equally difficult to follow. After all,

tobacco and alcohol are such intrinsic parts of our lives, even after the almost worldwide vilification of tobacco products after it was discovered that they caused cancer. It's not your fault if you can't decrease your intake of these products, but you need to realize that they are responsible for a lot of the damage that your body is suffering, as they introduce some of the most toxic chemicals into your body out of perhaps any other substances that we consume. If you are addicted to either cigarettes or alcohol, or if you feel as though they have become an unavoidable part of your social life, it's best not to quit cold turkey because you will just end up relapsing within a day or two, perhaps three if you have sufficient will power. The better option to pursue in this scenario is to gradually decrease the quantity that you consume. For example, if you generally drink four glasses of beer a day try decreasing the amount by one glass per week or even half a glass. The same technique can be used for cigarettes as well. Interestingly, although caffeine is a stimulant, it's actually an important part of your detox diet as you will see in list entry number 9.

Complete avoidance of all processed and chemically altered foods: Another no brainer, but this one should be relatively easy to accomplish at least when compared to the one before it. However, don't think that just because the media doesn't tell you they're bad doesn't mean that you don't get addicted to foods that have been processed or chemically altered. These foods positively affect your mood similar to the way very mild drugs do, and your body can get used to that. However, working these foods out of your daily life is fairly simple. The first thing you need to do, of course, is to cut out all fast food and just eating out in general. Cook food at home, make sure that the ingredients you use aren't processed and don't contain any chemical additives and you'll be good to go. You'll even really like this new diet of yours because it will begin to taste so good once you start to enjoy the real flavors of food rather than chemicals that provide you with a false sense of taste! Soda might be more difficult to quit since it is very addictive but using the same tactic you used with alcohol or cigarettes will definitely get the job done.

An increase in the intake of vegetables and fruits: Out goes the bad, in goes the good, this is the basic rule of any detox diet worth its salt and any detox diet that does not encourage this mindset will never be anything more than a hoax! The good that must go in is mostly fruits and vegetables based. Out of all of the foods that you can possibly eat, none are better for you than vegetables or fruits because they have absolutely everything that you could possibly want from your food! From vitamins to minerals to fiber, even protein if you eat the right vegetables, fruits and vegetables should ideally be all that your detox diet consists of but even just making these foods a regular part of your regular meals will make a huge difference. This is because, apart from the aforementioned vitamins, minerals etc. that fruits and vegetables contain, they also contain antioxidants. Antioxidants are chemicals that detoxify your body and get rid it of pretty much all of the toxic chemicals that are making it such an inefficient and unhealthy place. This means that the more fruits and vegetables you eat, the faster you will detoxify! Just don't overdo it because too much of anything can never be good.

A decrease in the intake of meat: Meat is an important part of the modern diet. The vast majority of people that are living in today's modern day and age incorporate a large amount of meat into their diets, to the point where the average modern meal is based around a meat related entree, with vegetables serving as side dishes and fruits little more than oft forgotten after thoughts. We can't really be blamed for this, after all meat tastes so good! However, red meat especially can clog up your system because it has a lot of saturated fat which is a chemical that can become quite toxic if you consume too much of it. Kicking the meat habit will be incredibly difficult, but as long as you cut down on red meat, reducing it to one serving a day, you will be able to detox your body successfully, as long as your fruit and vegetable intake is comparably high. If you quit meat, you can use nuts in order to supplement your protein intake. You can derive your entire daily requirement of protein entirely from nuts and legumes, which will allow you to stay healthy, possibly bulk up, and avoid saturated fats altogether!

Start buying organic: The way we grow foods has become increasingly warped. There was once a time when farming was just that: farming. Some crops were lost, some grew bad, but most grew normally and these crops were both delicious and healthy. Nowadays, however, farming is done on an industrial scale, which means that the same old methods that farmers once used simply won't cut it anymore. Farming now involves the spraying of pesticides and insecticides in order to make sure that every single crop makes it and is harvested, and you can imagine how dangerous these chemicals are when consumed. Hence, while detoxing it is extremely important to buy organic fruits and vegetables, and even meat, because these foods will not have any chemicals used to treat them at any stage of the manufacturing process. The vegetables and fruits will not have been grown in chemically treated fertilizer, they would not have been sprayed with poison to prevent them from being lost to plague, and this means that you will not be filling your body with poisons while you are on this diet, giving your body time to heal itself.

Eat raw as much as possible: This rule is part of the "good comes in" half of the detox motto. There are some foods that absolutely cannot be eaten raw, foods like potatoes, eggs and, of course, meat. However, there are a lot more foods that absolutely can be eaten raw, including the vast majority of vegetables as well as practically every fruit in existence, and it is important to eat these foods raw as much as you can. This is because of a little known fact: cooking drains foods of its nutrients. It kills germs and other microbes, but the heat from cooking also kills organic matter such as vitamins that reduces the nutritional effectiveness of the food that you are eating. Cooking also kills antioxidants, which as you will remember from a few rules ago are instrumental in helping you detoxify your system as fast as possible. Hence, in order to get the maximum nutritional benefit from the detox foods that you are eating, eat them raw! Also, try to avoid food that needs to be cooked. It's not that it's bad for you, it's just that there is not better diet than a raw vegan diet, so try to follow this diet if you want extremely effective results!

Drink as much water as possible: Water is the key to life. We can survive for days without food, indeed after a while we can even forget our hunger because our survival response kicks in and starts using up fat to keep us alive. However, we cannot survive more than a day or two without water, and the time we spend without water will be nothing more than pure agony. There is an important reason why this is so, and that is that water powers our body in every single way possible. Every liquid substance in our body needs water to exist, water exists somewhere in the process of the creation of that substance, from blood to bile to spit. Without water, these substances cannot replenish themselves. This means that your body will weaken and will be unable to fully utilize the detoxifying foods that you are eating. Additionally, water really cleans up your system in a meaningful and efficient way. Just like how it helps clean virtually everything, water

speeds up your metabolism and allows your body to use it to dilute the toxic substances within it to tolerable levels that makes them much easier to expel via excretion. The best way to increase your water intake is to replace your beverages with water. Instead of juice or soda, have water and get healthier for it!

Go for better grain choices: The types of grain that we eat are incredibly important because grains are not immune to the immense refinement that undergoes practically every type of food that we eat. The bread that we eat is usually made of refined flour that is what allows it to possess its white color and firm and consistent texture and shape. Real bread is supposed to be lumpy, it's supposed to be rough, in essence it's supposed to be exactly what it is: *real* bread. If you want to avoid toxic chemicals that would make you feel terrible by clogging up your entire system, the best thing that you can do is to avoid refined grains. Whether it's pasta or bread or any other food that is derived from a grain, make sure it's made from whole grain. Try to get bread that is as unprocessed as possible. Really, the only process that should go into the making of your bread is the baking itself, without which the bread wouldn't really be bread at all!

Drink coffee and tea in moderation: This may come across as somewhat odd considering the fact that stimulants are supposed to be bad for you. However, it is not the stimulants themselves but the chemicals they often bring with them that cause the harm. Nicotine, for example, is not that bad, but the cigarettes that are used to consume it contain tar and cyanide, two chemicals that you really don't want inside your body. Caffeine is actually not bad for you at all, the only real damage that it can do is upset your circadian rhythm and interrupt your sleep patterns, along with potentially getting you addicted to the point where you can't really get up without it. However, coffee and tea also possess antioxidants, and plenty of them. Tea especially is an enormous source of antioxidants, so try to consume it when you can. However, don't overdose on either of these beverages because the side effects, such as jitteriness and insomnia, are nothing to sneeze at!

Find alternates to dairy products: Dairy products are such a widely accepted part of our lives that we can barely even imagine a situation where drinking milk was not really good for your health. To be fair, milk is a great source of calcium and vitamin D, and is especially important in children that are in their growing phase. However, cow's milk is often treated using chemicals, and it is nearly impossible to get cow's milk that has not been chemically treated. Indeed, cow's milk that has not been treated is actually not safe to drink. Additionally, cow's milk is not designed for human consumption, and so our digestive system doesn't really agree with it. While you are on your detox diet, go for soymilk instead. It is better for your digestive system, can be found without any chemical treatment and is chock full of antioxidants to help you flush out the toxic chemicals from your body!

Chapter 10:

When is Detoxing Necessary?

In order to understand in which situations detoxification becomes necessary, one must first understand what exactly detoxification is supposed to accomplish. This helps provide a more balanced understanding of the subject that is very important while moving forward with the detoxification process.

Detoxification, through its removal of toxic substances from your body, improves your health, this much is true, but what it also does is that it helps you overcome some of your most destructive addictions.

This is because when your body becomes used to the toxic substances it now has within it, mostly due to the fact that these chemicals make it feel good, you become addicted to certain substances.

This means that detoxification pertains not just to specific diets intended to purge your body of toxins, it also refers to processes by which you can kick habits and addictions.

Cigarette Addiction

One example of a detoxification process is when you stop smoking. Your body has become so used to the nicotine that it has started to consider tar and cyanide to be feel good chemicals as well, which means that when you quit smoking you are going to feel certain symptoms These symptoms are called withdrawal. It is when your body is so dependent on certain drugs that it considers these substances to be healthy parts of what it needs in order to function properly. This means that when you quit cigarettes, you are going to experience withdrawal.

Certain symptoms of withdrawal include a loss of appetite, insomnia, irritability and just a general distaste for everything because all you want from your life while you are detoxing from cigarettes is, well, a cigarette. Quitting cold turkey is very possible, but bear in mind that it is going to be a somewhat uncomfortable process particularly if you are not especially strong willed.

Cigarette smoking is one of the most prevalent addictions in the world, despite the fact that it is widely known that smoking cigarettes will almost certainly cause cancer, whether in the lungs or in the mouth, in the long run. This goes to show just how incredibly addictive the stuff is, and how difficult it is to quit it.

Smoking becomes a part of our social gatherings, it becomes a part of how we bond with our bosses, becomes a part of how we deal with stress and anxiety in general. A large amount of people in the world, when faced with a problem that causes stress or seems insurmountable, deal with the situation right after they have smoked a cigarette and calmed their nerves.

However, when you quit smoking you will find that your overall health will start to appreciate considerably. Your lung capacity will increase as will your stamina, you will probably be able to become a lot more sexually active, your body will start absorbing nutrients in a much more efficient way and just in general you will start feeling a lot better than you did while you were smoking.

This is because your body recognizes that tar and cyanide are poisonous but ignores their presence due to the fact that they bring nicotine with them. Once you stop giving your body nicotine, it will start to clean house automatically by purging itself of all of these toxic chemicals Hence, quitting cigarettes and allowing your body time to evacuate itself of the toxic chemicals is one example of detoxification. If you are addicted to cigarettes, even if the addiction consists of two or three a day at the moment, you need to detox in order to prevent sinking into deeper addiction.

Alcohol Addiction

There are few substances in the world that are as destructive as alcohol. It is immensely addictive, and the worst part is that it is socially accepted as well which means that it is very easy to fall into the trap of alcohol addiction.

There is a limit to how much alcohol is acceptable. Having a beer or two, a glass of wine or a glass of whiskey while you are out with friends is alright because it does not introduce so much of the stuff that when you stop it would cause withdrawal.

However, when you start drinking every single day you will find that that is the start of a slippery slope that is very difficult to climb back up from. Doing anything every day gives your body the impression that it is a part of your daily diet and it slowly becomes dependent on that chemical.

What alcohol dependency does is that it makes you unable to deal with anxiety or stress without it. Additionally, people that are addicted to alcohol find that they are also unable to go to sleep without having a drink or two.

If you get to this point, you can be sure that you are on that slippery slope to alcohol addiction. However, frequent detoxes can help you ensure that you do not become dependent on alcohol because your body will be used to long periods where you do not consume the substance.

That is all an alcohol detox is really. An extended period of time where you do not consume any form of alcohol, whether at a party or at night in order to sleep. If you feel as though you are unable to cope with your emotions without alcohol, you probably have an addiction.

Keep in mind that a detox from alcohol would only really work if you drink at most four beers, two glasses of wine or a glass of whiskey every day. Any more than that and you are almost certainly addicted and will be unable to detox cold turkey without causing severe discomfort to yourself.

This is mostly due to the fact that your body has probably become utterly independent on the substance. Hence, if you drink a drink or two a day, go for the detox. If it's more than that, get yourself into alcoholics anonymous.

Drug Addiction

Addiction to drugs is one of the most severe epidemics in recent history. Ever since the invention of hardcore, refined drugs such as heroin and crystal meth, the amount of drug addicts has massively increased in recent times, to the point where millions of people are now addicted to hard drugs.

Hard drugs are not the only things that people are getting addicted to. Medicines that are often prescribed to people by their own doctors can be considered incredibly addictive due to the immense amounts of serotonin that they release within your brain in order to have their effect.

Drugs such as oxycodone, hydrocodone, vicodin and especially morphine, the unaltered and legal version of heroin, are incredibly addictive, and it should come as no surprise to you that all of these drugs are pain killers. Painkillers are, after all, placebos that give your brain a positive buzz to focus on instead.

This often happens when people are prescribed with painkillers following a surgery or an injury of some kind that has left them with pain. Doctors often give their patients an unlimited supply of these painkillers in order to help them deal with the pain that they are feeling.

However, this has the effect of making these people dependent on the drug, with the dependence working much in the same way that alcohol dependence does. When people get off the painkillers, they are sometimes unable to deal with pain at all because they are so used to using the painkillers to dull the sensation.

Hence, a lot of people end up addicted to these powerful painkillers and experience symptoms of withdrawal if they are not able to continue using these drugs. In this way an addiction is born, a process of detoxification becomes necessary.

Our body needs to learn how to deal with pain naturally again, which means that we need to rid it of all of these toxins in order to teach it to do that once more. The detox procedure works in exactly the same way, you just stop taking the drug entirely until you no longer need it.

However, in cases where you are addicted to heroin, crystal meth or have a severe dependence on prescription drugs, trying to quit cold turkey would end up causing you severe discomfort. Indeed, trying to completely stop using hard drugs such as heroin after you have developed a dependency for them can even result in your death, so it is important that you proceed with caution. If you feel as though you are dependent to a dangerous degree on these drugs, go and see a therapist and try your best to get yourself into narcotics anonymous.

In situations where the number of times you have tried hard drugs is still in the single digits, or situations where your use of prescription drugs is starting to or has recently started to get out of control, going on a detox and avoiding the substance can be the best way to get past your growing addiction.

Fast Food Addiction

An addiction to fast food is not usually what people have in mind when they picture addictions. However, fast food addictions are even more prevalent than drug addictions, and are extremely dangerous for one's health even if there is no chance of dying because of an overdose caused by fast food.

Fast food addiction is real because it is not normal food. Fast food is mass produced and heavily altered by chemicals in order to make it taste unnaturally good which helps our bodies ignore the fact that it is almost entirely junk which holds little to no nutritional value for our bodies.

These chemicals trigger a response in your brain that is shockingly similar to the one you get from consuming moderate level drugs. Your brain begins releasing dopamine and serotonin, two chemicals called the "feel good" chemicals because they are released whenever your body is doing anything that makes you feel pleasure.

This results in your body associating unhealthy fast food with a reward response within your brain and begins to crave it in increasing amounts. Nowadays, it is not uncommon for the average family to eat out two or three times a week. Certain people even eat fast food every single day, and there is a special group of people which certain fast food giants like to call "super heavy users" who eat more than one meal a day at a fast food place.

An addiction to fast food is incredibly dangerous because of the low nutritional value that fast food holds. Little to no vitamins or minerals, often not nearly enough fiber or carbohydrates and definitely no antioxidants whatsoever make fast food a terrible way to eat. What fast food does have are copious amounts of saturated fat, processed sugar in spades and protein since all fast food is basically meat.

Eating such a toxic cocktail of chemicals can result in obesity and diabetes, not to mention high cholesterol and blood pressure, heart palpitations, sleep apnea and the occasional heart attack. Regularly eating fast food is a recipe for death and nothing else, and harms you just as much in the long run as hard drugs even though the short term effects are not as severe.

Quitting fast food is a lot easier than quitting hard drugs or alcohol, however. The level of addiction has not yet reached the point where foodaholics anonymous has become a thing, and we should all be thankful for that, and so quitting fast food cold turkey will probably not cause you any real pain.

However, you should keep in mind that quitting fast food would cause certain withdrawal symptoms such as depression and sexual dysfunction. This is because your body is used to a mild high that you get after eating fast food and would crave it. However, you will not experience any severe form of discomfort and your health will improve within a few weeks of having quit fast food. Indeed, within days of quitting the stuff you won't even remember why you liked it so much.

Fast food addiction is a serious issue, and detoxing from these poisonous and toxic foods is essential if we want to improve our overall health and make for ourselves a brighter future.

Once your body is no longer addicted to fatty foods and sugary drinks you will feel your energy levels going up and will feel fresher throughout the day, all thanks to the fact that you detoxed from fast food in the first place.

The aforementioned addictions can all be treated to some extent using a process of detoxification. As long as your drug addiction is not too severe, quitting cold turkey is the best way to allow your body to rid itself of the chemicals that it has accumulated over the course of an unhealthy life.

Detoxing also tells you an important thing about yourself: it allows you to ascertain whether you are addicted or not. If you smoke on occasion or fairly regularly, if you drink every day, if you eat at a fast food place very often, even if you partake in hard drugs from time to time, you might be telling yourself that you are not addicted, that you can quit absolutely any time you want.

Detoxing is the way you can put yourself to the test. Try to go without your choice of drug for three days and your body will tell you if you are addicted or not. If you are unable to deal with stress or anxiety or start suffering from insomnia, you can be sure that you are addicted. If you start experiencing withdrawal symptoms, your detox will have told you something extremely important about the things that you are addicted to.

Chapter 11:

When Can Detoxing Be Dangerous?

The people doing the detoxing rather than the process of detoxing itself cause the dangers of detoxing most often. Remember, detoxing is a natural process whereby you purge your body of dangerous substances and toxins in order to help it function in a more efficient manner and improve your overall health.

However, much like any good tool, detoxing must be used in a proper manner. There are detox diets out there that are endorsed by big name celebrities, celebrities who probably don't use these diets themselves and are just doing the endorsements for the money that could cause some major damage to body.

Also, there is such a thing as "too much of a good thing". Detoxing too much can be dangerous as well, particularly if detoxing involves overdosing on a single food that supposedly helps in the detox process and ignoring all of the other equally important areas of your nutrition that you begin to neglect. Doing so will result in nutritional deficiencies which can develop into serious problems if they are not addressed.

In order to help you detox in a safer manner, here are some ways in which detoxing can become dangerous:

> Restriction of nutrients: Certain detox diets encourage you to avoid certain nutrients because they supposedly cause a buildup of toxic chemicals within your system. You need to keep in mind that toxic chemicals are not caused by the consumption of nutrients. Nutrients are just what they are, nutrients, and toxic

chemicals and nutrients are never the same thing. Avoiding certain nutrients can cause severe problems such as malnutrition. You are going on a detox diet to improve your health, and avoiding any kind of nutrient will be detrimental to your health in some way or another.

Restriction of calories: A lot of detox diets encourage you to lower your calorie intake. There is absolutely no reason that you have to do this. Reducing one's intake of calories is important if you want to lose weight, not if you want to detoxify your body. Reducing calorie intake can result in deterioration of your health, especially if it's done to an extreme extent to the point where you are going hours without eating. This is actually the opposite of what you should actually be doing.

Liquid based diets: These diets are another example of what is wrong with the industry that has been built around detox diets. A thing that is meant to improve people's health is now being used to earn money, but such is the way of the world and there is little we can do about it apart from learn to avoid these diets. Liquid diets can be extremely dangerous for your health because liquid foods don't provide the same fiber content and nutritional value as solid foods and liquid diets virtually never provide enough protein. Hence, avoiding liquid diets is the best way for you to keep your health sound while detoxing. Make a special effort to avoid diets that encourage you to consume only water, as these diets will completely wreck your system and severely lower the quality of your health.

Shortcut diets: There is no such thing as a shortcut to good health, and any diet that is using that line to coax you into buying it is definitely not worth your time. Such products are a part of the problem, actually, because they put it into people's minds that the process of detoxing can be accomplished within an extremely short span of time and thus is not worth investing a lot of time into. These diets also involve a lot of shortcuts such as calorie counting that makes you lose weight and thus would make you feel as though you are detoxing. Remember, detoxing has absolutely nothing to do with weight. It is supposed to flush your body of internal toxins and help make you feel good. It will make your skin glow but it is certainly not supposed to make you lose weight, so if a diet offers you a shortcut to getting a clean internal system, avoid that diet like the plague.

Diets that aren't detox diets at all: Detoxing has become the name of a product now that companies have wizened up to the fact that detox diets are incredibly effective and are thus become incredibly popular, especially in recent times. However, these companies don't know the first thing about what a detox diet is supposed to do, they assume that it is just like any other diet and is supposed to make you lose weight. Hence, avoid these diets that big name companies offer you. In essence, this rule is an amalgamation of all of the rules before it. Detoxing is supposed to be relaxing and help you feel good, not make you sick!

Now that you have gotten a general idea of what kinds of detox procedures can be dangerous, you also need to keep in mind the previous chapter. Detoxing from hard drugs can be extremely dangerous, especially if you have become dependent on the drug.

In fact, detoxing from drugs by quitting outright all of a sudden could even result in death. Detoxing from alcohol can be similarly dangerous, as it can cause symptoms of withdrawal that would feel similar to an illness and would almost certainly result in you being out of commission for a period of time.

Now it is time for you to understand the various symptoms that come with detoxing dangerously. Most of these symptoms come about as a result of detoxing too quickly due to the fact that you are consuming too many foods that aid in the detox process.

You might also be detoxing improperly, usually due to the fact that you are following an improper diet of some kind. Whatever the case may be, if you experience any of the following symptoms you will know that you are detoxing improperly in some way and should revert back to your normal diet.

Hair loss: Certain diets force you to leave certain nutrients out of your overall diet. These diets have been mentioned in this chapter before and should be avoided. A sign that you are not receiving enough nutrients is if you start to lose hair. This is a very extreme sign of malnutrition, and if you start experiencing abnormal hair loss during your detox diet stop detoxing immediately, revert to your original diet and preferably go see a doctor.

Skin irritation: This is another sign that you are running low on certain nutrients. Skin irritation is actually a normal part of detoxing, but if the irritation results in major breakage in your skin, in essence if the irritation is severe, then you are detoxing improperly and should stop immediately. However, if the skin irritation that you are facing is mild, for example a breakout of acne for a short period of time, then you have nothing whatsoever to worry about. Additionally, if you see red or pink patches on your skin during your detox period don't worry, as this is completely normal.

General irritability: You might start feeling cranky or irritable while you are on your detox diet. This is normal to a degree, as your body is craving the feel good chemicals that it was once able to get so easily and is now being deprived of. However, if your irritability turns into hostility, for example if you start experiencing violent mood swings, you will need to end your detox diet immediately. Improper detoxing can cause hormonal imbalances that can result in these sudden shifts in your mood.

Nausea or fever: A certain amount of nausea is to be expected while you are detoxing. Your body is getting rid of toxic chemicals that it has within it and this induces a feeling of nausea within you. However, vomiting is never supposed to happen while you are detoxing, and neither is fever. If either of these things happen to you while you are detoxing it means that your detox diet is improper and will result in a deterioration of your health. You are probably low on some kind of nutrient or are consuming too much detox food that is not agreeing with your body.

Weakness: While you are detoxing you can expect to feel a little lazy while the detox diet progresses. This is because your body has lost something that used to motivate it a lot. However, a detox diet is under no circumstances supposed to cause weakness in any form. If you begin feeling weak while you are on your detox diet, it probably means that you are not consuming enough calories which is resulting in your body being low on glucose and going into starvation mode. If you feel weak during your detox diet, try eating more while you are on it or stop in entirely.

Heart palpitations: Heart palpitations are a serious sign that something is wrong. They are not a normal part of detox diets in any way, and if you experience an irregular heartbeat you can rest assured that your detox diet is definitely not working out for you. Certain detox diets cause a deficiency in electrolytes that are necessary to keep the heart pumping efficiently and regularly. Go to a doctor and ask them if this was caused by a preexisting condition. If it wasn't, you need to change your diet immediately.

Depression: A little mood of depression is to be expected while you are detoxing because your body is so used to getting chemically induced shots of happiness hormones in its brain. It forgets how regulate the levels of serotonin and dopamine on its own, which means that for the first few days depression is normal. However, if it stretches on for more than four days, or if the depression gets extremely severe, you need to go see a doctor immediately. Ascertain the cause of the depression, and if it is being caused by your detox diet you will need to end it immediately.

Abdominal pain: There is absolutely no situation where abdominal pain is a normal part of a good detox diet. Abdominal pain is actually the opposite of what you should be feeling. Detox diets sometimes result in diarrhea, but this only lasts for a day or two at mist. If it lasts for longer, or if you start feeling any kind of abdominal pain, stop the diet immediately. You have probably become deficient in iron and fiber due to the nature of the particular diet that you are following, and continuing with the diet might end up causing irreparable damage to your digestive system.

Sore eyes: This is another sign that the diet that you are following is not quite right for you. Much like many of the other entries on this list, sore eyes are not, in fact, part of a normal detox diet. They are actually a sign that something dangerous is going on in your body caused by a deficiency in some nutrient or the other, more often than not this nutrient being vitamin C. If your eyes start becoming sore while you are on your detox diet, end the diet immediately, revert back to your original diet and go see a doctor immediately.

Constant drowsiness: As has been mentioned in a previous entry in this list, a little bit of laziness is a normal part of a detox diet as your body feels lethargic without the chemicals that made it feel so good. However, if you start feeling constantly drowsy you can be sure that the diet that you are is not good for you and that you should revert back to your original diet. Constant drowsiness can be the result of a hormonal imbalance or it can be the result of an unnecessarily low calorie intake. Either way, avoiding the diet that causes such a symptom is best.

Lowered immunity to disease: Another sign that your detox diet is absolutely not working for you is if you start getting sick a lot during the diet. Detox diets are never supposed to weaken your immune system, so if you start getting sick you can be sure that the diet you are following is not quite right. In general, if you can trace the origin of your sicknesses to the starting of your detox diet then you have definitely adopted a diet that is decidedly bad for you and should be changed if you don't want your health to deteriorate further.

Dizziness: Slight light headedness can be considered a normal part of the detox experience as your body is still getting used to functioning without all of those drugs and chemicals being poured into it. However, if you get so dizzy that you lose your balance you're in trouble. Detox diets are not supposed to have a profound effect on your balance, so unless you have a preexisting condition you should stop following your diet immediately and go see a doctor. Dizziness could be the result of a low consumption of calories, an extension of the aforementioned weakness, and should be taken seriously.

How Does Detoxing Help?

Now that you have come to learn about all of the dangers of detoxing, you are probably a little afraid to start detoxing yourself. After all, why would anyone attempt to do anything that could cause them so much harm?

The thing you need to realize is that all of the aforementioned dangers and negative symptoms are the result of improper detoxing, detoxing that involves unnecessary limitations on nutritional intake and forces you to abandon important parts of your diet. Such diets should be viewed as the opposite of what actual detoxing is supposed to do.

Yes, detoxing properly will actually have the complete opposite of all of the negative effects that have been mentioned in the previous chapter. In the worst case scenarios, you will get a taste of the milder negative symptoms, like skin irritation, and then your body will become accustomed to the chemical free way in which you are now living your life.

Hence, it is important to understand that detoxing is more about the good than the bad. All you need to do is to follow the proper ways in which you can detox, and you will be able to enjoy the following marvelous benefits:

> Better breath: Bad breath is one of the worst social faux pas that one can commit. It can put off dates, make people think less of you and just, in general, ruin your social life. This is probably even more frustrating for people when they realize that their bad breath is not even their fault! For some people, no matter how much they brush and how much mouthwash that they use, they simply can't get rid of their bad breath. This is actually because their colon is backed up. This is a little known cause of bad breath that actually has nothing to do with oral hygiene. Going on a detox diet clears out your colon if it is backed up, which will actually make your breath smell better once the diet is over. However, while the diet is ongoing remember that detox diets often cause bad breath. This is because the toxins are being expelled from your body and obviously are not going to smell very good! This is a normal part of the detoxing process, so just keep a breath mint or two handy and you'll be good to go.

> Alleviation of your chronic diseases: Chronic diseases are perhaps some of the most difficult things that people have to endure. They are lifelong companions, and rough ones at that, and living with them for a long time does tend to take its toll. Chronic illnesses can actually have a deep impact on your life, forcing you to adopt

different habits and in some ways can become a hindrance to your social life as well, especially if your chronic disease is particularly debilitating. However, if you detox properly you can actually reduce the symptoms of your chronic illnesses to the point where you will be able to live a completely normal life! Our chronic diseases may be caused by genetic anomalies but they are usually greatly exacerbated by the environment we surround ourselves in. The food we eat and the beverages we drink have a huge effect on the way our bodies handle these chronic illnesses. If you detox, you are freeing your body of toxins. These toxins that were clogging up your system force your body to handle them rather than your illness. Once they are flushed out, your body will be able to focus on its chronic problems instead, thereby making your symptoms a lot more bearable!

Enhancement of your immune system: This is partially tied to the previous amazing benefit that you receive from detoxing properly. Our immune system is what keeps us alive, it is an interconnected system of checks and balances that starts at our skin and is able to fight infections and diseases for a good long while, allowing us to live in the world without fear. However, our immune systems have recently started to become quite weak. This is mostly due to the creation of modern medicine. Modern medicine has slowly started to replace the work our immune system does with medicines which do the immune system's job for it. This is not to say that modern medicine doesn't save lives, it is an important part of why disease is so uncommon, only that we are becoming dependent on medicines. Detoxing allows you to boost your immune system by ridding your body of the substances that were getting in its way. The chemicals we consume make our already weakening immune system even more sluggish. By purging these chemicals, we allow our immune system to work at full capacity.

Weight loss: this may come as a surprise to you, particularly after previous chapters in which it is stated that weight loss is not what detox diets are for. This is actually true. The purpose of detox diets is never to lose weight, it is to purge your body of harmful chemicals. You should never start a detox diet with the intention of losing weight because that will warp the way that you approach the diet and might cause problems in the long run if you start to use detoxing incorrectly because you want it to make you lose weight. That being said, if you approach detoxing correctly and apply it with all of the correct rules and specifications, you will find that you will start to lose weight after a week or two of being on the diet. This is mostly because your metabolism gets stronger after the toxins have been flushed from your body, which means that your body can spend more time on metabolizing food without those toxins slowing it down. Additionally, the foods that you eat while you are on your detox diet are actually naturally not fatty or sugary, and thus allow you to lose weight while you are following this diet.

Slows down the aging process: We are living longer in today's modern day and age, thanks to modern medicine and its miracles, but at the same time we are aging quite quickly as well. This is simply due to the fact that the chemicals that we are consuming on a daily basis are simply toxic and are forcing our organs, especially our skin, to endure a lot more wear and tear than they would have otherwise. The things that we consume also contain a large amount of heavy metals as well as free radicals, both of which contribute heavily to the aging process. Detoxing, naturally, rids our bodies of these free radicals as well as these heavy metals that are polluting our systems, thereby allowing us to significantly slow down the aging process and prevent us from looking like we are forty when we are just thirty. This might just be a deal breaker for a lot of people considering the vain and vapid society that we currently live in which values physical beauty over anything else. Detoxing allows you to stay young while at the same time maintaining your youth in a natural and holistic way. It also doesn't hurt that detoxing can be considered a much, much cheaper alternative to all of these procedures that people go through in order to stay young.

Makes you feel better: We eat the things we eat and consume the things that we consume and throughout all of this consumption we do not realize that the joy that we are feeling is fleeting and temporary. The feeling of contentment we get after eating fast food is caused by the chemical makeup of that food, by the fact that the food has been specifically designed in order to make it stimulate the pleasure center of the brain. This is why we are never truly satisfied while we are living that lifestyle. We constantly crave another hit, no matter what it is that we are addicted to. Detoxing allows you to break that cycle. You feel true joy when your body is free of all chemicals and foreign toxins and is feeling the way it should feel. All of the joint pains and aches, all of the chronic diseases we develop, all of these go away when we detoxify our bodies because it is these toxins that were causing these problems in the first place!

Improves your energy: There are a large number of people out there whose number one complaint would be that they simply don't have enough energy throughout the day. They are unable to get up in the morning without drinking coffee, are unable to get through the day without some kind of stimulant that will help them gain enough energy to do the things that they need to do. This is mostly because of the toxins that have been built up inside them. These toxins prevent energy from being used efficiently by our bodies, which means that when you detox you are going to be discovering a whole fount of energy within you that you had never tapped before. Once the toxins are out of your body, your body will be able to process the foods that you are eating a lot more efficiently, it will be able to regulate your sleep patterns in a more efficient manner as well. You will find that you won't need to sleep as much, but while you do sleep it will be like a rock, and when you wake up you will be so fresh that you won't even need coffee or any of the other supplements that you had made a part of your morning kick start.

Improves your skin: This is an example of one of the negative things that could happen if you follow your detox diet improperly going absolutely right if you properly follow your detox diet with all of the rules and specifications that have been put in place in order to make it effective. If you follow a bad detox diet your skin will probably break out in acne and rashes and they simply won't go away until you stop following your diet. If you follow a proper detox diet, the result will actually be the same for the first couple of days. While your body is ridding itself of these toxins your skin might break in acne or rashes, but after they go away your skin will be positively glowing. All of the good things that you would have been putting into your system during your detox diet as well as all of the toxins that would be evacuating your body during this time would result in your skin clearing up, becoming naturally smooth and overall becoming the best skin without you having to resort to expensive beauty products.

Improved mental state: Eating all of these weird chemicals and substances definitely has an effect on your mental state. These chemicals alter the levels of chemicals in your brain, after all, so it can be assumed that your brain loses the ability to regulate itself. It becomes dependent on the fast food and drugs that you consume in order to boost its mood, and so it floods itself with depressant chemicals in order to balance your mental state out. However, since you cannot be eating fast food literally every second of the day, this probably gets you depressed and gives you a negative emotional and mental state. When you detoxify yourself, you will be depressed for a few days, but after this phase is ended you will feel absolutely fantastic, as though the world were at your feet. Your improved mental state will be the result of your brain being able to regulate its level of chemicals itself without the outside influence of the chemicals brought in by fast food, cigarettes or alcohol. Overall, detoxification allows you to feel like yourself again, and when it's over you will feel as though a fog has been lifted!

Chapter 12:
Other Ways to Detoxify

There is a misconception regarding what exactly detoxification is. Many people seem to think that detoxification involves following a strict diet where you are forbidden from eating certain kinds of food whereas other kinds of food you are strictly required to eat.

However the reality of the matter is actually much different. Detoxification does not quite require you to go on a diet. Rather it is more about avoiding the foods and drugs that make your body full of toxins and substances that slow it down and prevent it from doing the things it needs to do to keep you functioning.

Hence, it often comes as a surprise to people when they find out that there are several ways that they can detoxify their body without even having to alter their diets or change the way they eat in any significant way. In fact, these ways are often just as if not more effective than the detox diets that have become so popular as of late.

The main thing to remember with the following methods is that moderation is key. None of these methods are diets, and most of them require you to only change very minor details about your lifestyle.

Saunas

What a lot of people don't know about the detox process has a lot to do with the fact that they don't know much about how their body works. People think that toxins within their body are black swathes of sludge that cover their organs and arteries.

However, these toxins are actually not quite like that. They are actually trace chemicals that are in the blood stream, which means that they are a lot more insidious than a lot of people seem to understand because they are so difficult to pin point and tackle, which makes a lot of people think that altering the diet is the only way to go about expelling these substances.

However, there is another way to expel these toxins from your body, and that is through your sweat. When you sweat, your body removes all of the impurities that are just beneath your skin. Interestingly, this is where most of the toxins that we consume end up being deposited; just beneath our skin.

When we sweat, these impurities, the toxins that we are trying to get rid of, are expelled from our bodies without us even having to alter our diets in any way. Saunas are, therefore, one of the best ways to detoxify your body, particularly if you are looking for quick results. Try to go into the sauna for half an hour about three to five days per week.

Exercise

We are not a dumb species in general. We know what's good for us and what isn't, what we should do and what we shouldn't. We are more than aware of what we need to do in order to live long and healthy lives happily and without worry. Yet we do not pursue these options, we choose to fill our bodies with poison simply because they provide us with momentary pleasure.

This is probably why we usually avoid exercising. We know that it is good for us, we know that it can help make us a lot healthier, but we choose not to do it. However, it is important to note just how amazing exercise truly is.

Exercise is not just a way to lose weight quickly and in healthy amounts, it's not just a way to get healthier and stronger and to live a longer life. Exercise is one of the most effective ways to detox your body as well.

When we exercise, our body pumps blood and oxygen a lot faster because we need it. It is forced to work a lot more efficiently than it usually has to. This makes it efficient, but more importantly it also makes you sweat.

As you probably read under the previous subheading in this chapter, sweating really helps you to detox. Exercise is an even better way to sweat because the vigorously pumping blood is purified, allowing you to expel even more toxins than you would have been able to had you just sat there in the sauna.

Lemon water

As had been said just before this list of small things you can do to detox your body started, the most important things that we do in order to detox are often small. These involve tiny changes to the way we live our lives that help our bodies in enormous ways to flush the toxins out from within themselves.

One of these small things that you can do in order to help your body detoxify itself is to drink lemon water. Lemons are one of the most amazing fruits in existence. They contain copious amounts of vitamin C, and they are also chock full of antioxidants which, as you will probably remember from one of the previous chapters, is one of the best substances that you can have if you want to detoxify your body as they dissolve and weaken the toxic chemicals.

Vitamin C also increases a compound in the liver that greatly helps its job and helps to detoxify your body even further. It also doesn't hurt that water is possibly one of the most important detox drinks in the world because nothing else is quite as effective as water when it comes to diluting toxic chemicals and helping make the whole detoxification process easier for your body.

Try to drink all of your water with a bit of lemon in it. If not, try to have a couple of glasses of lemon infused water first thing in the morning and see just how well the rest of your day goes!

Avoid dairy

Dairy has always been considered the staple drink if you want to get healthy. Throughout our youths we were told that if we drank milk we would grow up to be big and strong, and to an extent it is true that milk helps us to become healthier. It is an important source of vitamin D and calcium and helps to make bones stronger. It is particularly important for children who are growing.

However, milk is also quite detrimental to the detoxification process. Drinking milk facilitates the buildup of mucus and it also makes the liver slow down its activities. The liver is one of the most important organs in the entire detoxification process, and so anything that makes it less able to do the important job that it does must be cut out.

Simply removing milk from your diet will help your body start to detoxify itself automatically. This may seem somewhat difficult, particularly considering that dairy products are such an important part of our ever day diets in this modern day and age, but if you really work at it you will find that it's actually not that difficult at all.

There are so many new options out there to traditional dairy products that you will soon find that you don't miss it at all. Soy milk as well as soy cheese are excellent alternatives to regular dairy products and don't clog up your liver at all!

Cut out the alcohol

We consume a lot of poisonous substances in our day to day lives. They make us feel good, help us to function in a lot of ways, and it is almost shocking how incredibly dependent we have become on these substances. It is particularly surprising considering that none of these substances are important for our survival, yet they are both more valuable and more sought after than food.

Perhaps none of these substances is as poisonous, nor as widely desired and celebrated, as alcohol. Alcohol is, plain and simple, a poison. The way it makes us feel when we consume it is a mild form of poisoning. However, we drink it as though we need it to survive, and in many ways we do because our social interactions, our confidence, all of these things seem to require alcohol.

Alcohol is one of the most severe sources of the toxins in our body out of all of the other substances that we consume, and cutting it out is possibly the best way to begin detoxing. After all, the first step to detoxing is actually stopping the consumption of poisonous toxins in the first place. When you stop consuming these toxins, your body will be able to start removing the toxins that are already present within it.

This also works if you quit smoking cigarettes. Stop filling your body up with the substances that harm it and you will find that it will start to heal itself automatically.

Cupping

This is perhaps one of the least known methods of detoxification these days, but that does not mean that it is the newest. In fact, cupping is one of the oldest methods of detoxification known to man, being practiced in the orient for over two millennia before the concept of detoxing became popular in the west.

The procedure is, for lack of a better word, somewhat radical, but it is also immensely effective. It can only be performed by a trained professional and must in no circumstances be tried at home because of the delicacy of the whole endeavor.

If you opt for the procedure, an expert will make a small cut in your back and place a small glass bowl with a flame inside it over the cut. The flame will burn up all of the air inside the bowl, creating a vacuum that would suck in blood from the cut.

This procedure may sound disgusting and painful but it is actually only the former of those things. It is not painful at all, and it is only disgusting because the blood that comes out will actually be quite dark and murky because it is dirty blood full of all of the toxins that you have consumed over the course of your life.

This is an extremely effective way to ensure that all of the toxins are pulled from your body, and it involves absolutely no changes to your diet whatsoever. However, the delicacy of the whole procedure just goes to show how dangerous the procedure can be if the proper precautions are not taken.

As long as you get cupping done by a trained professional, there is absolutely no harm and a great deal of good that it can do to you. Additionally, remember that everything is good in moderation. Too much cupping can definitely be bad for you because it can result in unnecessary blood loss.

Dry Brushing

This technique can actually go hand in hand with the very first technique mentioned in this list that involved sweating in a sauna in order to get rid of the impurities that have become piled up within our systems.

Dry brushing is basically what the name says it is. It involves taking a firm brush and very gently brushing your dry skin with it. This stimulates your pores and helps make them more efficient at what they do best: removing the impurities from within your body.

There are special brushes that come at herbal stores that are actually optimized to help you dry brush your skin and help your pores really open up and breathe, allowing you to relax while your body does the detoxing for you. This is a great example of how you can detox without having to resort to changing your entire lifestyle.

The reason that this can work so well hand in hand with the sauna technique is that sloughing off your dead skin in the sauna will help the steam reach your pores in an even more effective way. This means that the impurities will come out in even more copious amounts than they would have otherwise.

All of this is about improving the effectiveness of your body's own, natural detoxification process. Your body wants to be clean, and if you just give it the chance it will do all of the hard work for you!

Chapter 13:
Foods That Help in the Detox Process

There are certain foods that you can eat in order to make the whole process of detoxing easier and more efficient. Certain foods seem as though they have been created for the sole purpose of facilitating proper detoxification, and these foods are just what the doctor ordered if you feel as though your body is unable to function properly because of the fact that it is overflowing with toxins.

These foods are actually very easy to buy, and are virtually all fruits and vegetables. Here is a list of these foods in alphabetical order:

Artichokes: As you can probably tell by the amount of times it was mentioned in the previous chapter, the liver is pretty important as far as the whole process of detoxification goes, and artichokes are possible the best vegetables that you can eat in order to improve the functioning of your liver. At the very least, artichokes are one of the most important vegetables that help in this department. The way it helps the liver is that helps it to produce more bile, a substance that your body needs in order to successfully detoxify itself in an efficient manner.

Apples: As the saying goes, "An apple a day keeps the doctor away". There is a very good reason that this saying has come about, and that reason is that apples are just incredibly healthy fruits. Within their mealy flesh they have vitamins and minerals, not to mention fiber that not a lot of fruits have as well as a number of phytochemicals. These phytochemicals are incredibly important in the whole detoxification process, and are what make the apple such an important part of any detoxification diet. Just eat an apple in the morning and you'll be good to go!

Almond: Vegetables have been covered now as have been fruits, now all that is left is the nut category, and what an important category it is! Almonds are the kings of nuts because they are incredibly high in a specific form of vitamin E that helps boost the body's ability to detoxify itself. Additionally, almonds contain copious amounts of calcium and protein as well as the healthy and unsaturated variety of fatty acids. All in all, almonds are pretty much a super food and having a handful of almonds in the morning can help you detox as well as really improve your memory!

Asparagus: although being universally reviled by children everywhere, the asparagus actually doesn't taste all that bad. Asparagus is also, incidentally, an incredibly healthy food to eat because of the wide variety of benefits that it provides. It prevents cancer, first and foremost, but in this context the most important benefit that it provides is that it helps to drain your liver. Often when the toxins in our body are too high, the liver is unable to detoxify and gets backed up. Asparagus helps alleviate this issue by draining the liver!

Avocadoes: Avocadoes might just be one of the most delicious vegetables that money can buy. They also happen to be detox powerhouses, being packed with antioxidants and nutrients that don't just detoxify your body, lower your cholesterol and help clean up clogged blood vessels as well! One of the most important roles that avocadoes play is that they help the liver detoxify the body in a very specific way. A lot of fast food comes packed with synthetic chemicals, something avocadoes actually help the liver to break down. Hence, avocadoes play an especially important role in the struggle for a toxin free body!

Basil: Basil is not exactly a vegetable. In fact, it is more of a spice or an herb, and it is one of the most important herbs that you can possibly add to your food. One of the most important roles that basil plays is that it helps to protect the liver. The liver would obviously be unable to detoxify the body if it was sick, which means in protecting the sole organ that can help the body become a toxin free place, basil plays a role that is unspeakably important and very rarely ever credited.

Beets: If there was one vegetable in the entire vegetable kingdom that could be called a powerhouse, it would the beet. If the artichoke is the king of all vegetables, then the beet is the knight, powerful and multitalented. They are chock full of phytochemicals which help your liver remove toxins from within your body. Additionally, beets have the added benefit of purifying blood themselves, which means that they are able to help the liver do its job and help lessen its workload as well. Since the liver is possibly one of the most overworked organs in our bodies, beets are nothing short of a godsend.

Blueberries: No breakfast treat can be complete without the sprinkling of delicious blueberries on waffles or pancakes. What makes them so special is that they are actually natural painkillers, and they don't just deaden pain they lessen inflammation as well! The nutrients present within blueberries are extremely important for the liver, as they are special nutrients called phytonutrients that are specifically meant to nourish the liver and provide it energy while it detoxifies the body. The liver needs helpers, but it needs nutrients as well otherwise it won't be able to function!

Brazil nuts: often considered one of the tastiest nuts around, Brazil nuts are also packed with selenium. Selenium is mostly known for being able to flush out excess amounts of mercury from our system, but a little known other use that our bodies have for selenium is as a bit of a medic for our poor liver. While the liver does battle with the toxins, the selenium from Brazil needs patch up its wounds and helps it to recover from the strain of having to work so hard to clean up a body that is so chock full of toxins!

Broccoli: broccoli has been ingrained in the minds of children everywhere as being a yucky vegetable, and this time even us adults would tend to agree most of the time, unlike with asparagus that is actually fairly tasty. However, broccoli is actually an essential part of the entire process of detoxification because it specifically works by aiding the enzymes created by your liver to help flush the toxins from our bodies. These enzymes work by diluting the power of these toxins, breaking them apart and making them easier for the liver to manage. Detoxification wouldn't be possible without broccoli!

Brussels sprouts: Brussels sprouts are once again not quite the most delicious vegetables on the planet. However, what they do not possess in taste they make up for by being extremely important to the whole process of detoxification. Brussels sprouts contain certain phytochemicals that are also present in broccoli. However, Brussels sprouts contain these in much, much larger quantities. So where broccoli helps in creating the enzymes that break the toxins down, Brussels sprouts give the body, and the liver in particular, ammo to help fight the toxins when they appear in their weakened forms after going through the enzymes.

Cabbage: This may seem like a list of vegetables that you never want to eat, but rest assured that each of these vegetables is here for a reason. Cabbage is especially notorious for making people gassy, but it has a good reason for doing this. After all, it boosts the whole process of digestion and makes it a lot more efficient.

Not only does cabbage contain important chemicals that help the liver detoxify the body, they also help the body to excrete all of these toxins. After all, once the liver is done breaking the toxins down and weakening them, they have to be excreted otherwise there will have been no point.

Cilantro: this vegetable is also known as coriander, and is often used as more of a garnishing rather than an actual vegetable that people actively eat. One of the most important roles that cilantro plays is that it helps to get certain extremely dangerous toxins out of the body, toxins that the liver can't handle. These toxins are heavy metals such as mercury that are very poisonous for the body. Cilantro is also chocked full of antioxidants making it an excellent choice for your detox diet!

Cinnamon: one of the most fragrant and aromatic spices around, cinnamon is also famous, or rather infamous, for the cinnamon challenge in which people realized that cinnamon was, despite its sweet taste, a spice after all. It is also one of the foods with the richest concentration of antioxidants in the entire world. Incorporating cinnamon into your everyday life, such as drinking it in tea or sprinkling it over cake, is an excellent way to greatly boost your daily intake of antioxidants. Cinnamon also gives you a good energy boost, which is a nice bonus considering how much it detoxifies your body!

Cranberries: apart from inspiring the name of a famous Welsh pop band, cranberries have become famous for being old people fruits. This is because they greatly help in the prevention of urinary tract infections and help make the whole process of urination a lot easier. Additionally, in the context of detoxing, cranberries are extremely important because they provide very specific phytochemicals that few easily available fruits provide which greatly help the liver break down toxins and chemicals and process it into urine. Cranberries also help the body to excrete the toxins much in the same way cabbage does.

Dandelions: flowers in general are not considered food, and a flower as dainty and as delicate as a dandelion would certainly never be considered so. However, dandelions are extremely helpful for the liver in its struggle to break down toxins in order to make them easy to excrete. Their specific and rather unique nutritional makeup enables them to be extremely helpful to the liver because they help to strain the blood and rid it of toxins and wastes. This means that eating dandelion leaves with your salad would make it easier for your liver to do its job, and if any organ in our body deserves a break from time to time it's our liver.

Fennel: fennel is uniquely important to the liver's struggle against toxins as well, much in the same way dandelions are although its nutrients serve a different purpose. It provides a B vitamin called folate that helps to convert certain specific but extremely dangerous substances into benign molecules that the body can excrete without causing itself any major harm. Since fennel is such a concentrated source of folate as well as a specific anti microbial variant of vitamin C, it should make up a large part of your overall diet.

Flaxseeds: there has been a recent surge in the popularity of flaxseeds after their benefits were made known to the general public. One of their most important functions is that they provide wonderful, wholesome fiber that is essential to allowing your digestive system to excrete properly. As you already known, once the liver is done breaking the toxins down into more manageable and less dangerous or completely benign compounds, all that is left is that the body must excrete these toxins. Flaxseeds allow the body to do this in a more efficient manner.

Garlic: a favorite vegetable of both Italian as well as Indian cuisines! Despite being so far apart, these cuisines both seem to understand the importance of garlic, all of which lies in the fact that it helps boost the immune system while providing invaluable aid in the liver's struggle to break down toxins and make them benign enough to excrete. One of the most important elements of garlic is, perhaps, sulfur, which helps the liver create enzymes and provides invaluable support especially after you have a large amount of junk food and the liver is backed up in its attempts to clean up your system.

Ginger: Ginger is another staple of Indian cuisine although it is not equally celebrated in Italian cuisine the way garlic is. Possibly the most important role that ginger plays is that it helps the liver to get leaner. This is important when you consider the fact that we eat a lot more fat than we need. The liver tends to get a buildup of fat around it as a result. A fatty liver is unable to do its job properly, which means that if not for ginger our livers would be unable to detoxify our bodies at all!

Goji berries: these berries could potentially prove to be an alternative to raisins, a far healthier version at that. Goji berries possess a large amount of beta carotene that the liver really needs in order to do its job. Additionally, it aids the whole process of detoxification by providing the body with an enormous amount of vitamins. It is an extremely important source of vitamin C, which incidentally is one of the most important vitamins when it comes to flushing your body of toxins. A regular supply of goji berries can help you get healthier in no time!

Grapefruit: grapefruit possesses what can arguably be considered the most startlingly beautiful flesh of any fruit in world. However, it is equally bitter, even though the beauty of its flesh would imply sweetness. Much like many other entries in this list, the grapefruit makes up for the fact that it does not taste very good by being extremely good for you. It possesses a chemical called lycopene that is instrumental in the fighting of free radicals. This helps your liver get into its peak form within no time, making grapefruit an important part of every diet.

Green tea: As has been mentioned before, tea can be considered an important part of any detox diet because they contain so many anti oxidants. However, there is no tea in the world that has as many antioxidants as green tea. This is simply due to the fact that green tea is the least processed tea in the world. The leaves are almost exactly the way they were in the wild, all you do is boil them and drink the tea. The health benefits that green tea provides are massive, and the amount of help that the liver receives from it is similarly sized.

Hemp: Again, this food is yet another addition to the foods in this list that cannot be considered particularly tasty, however hemp is also one of the healthiest foods in the world. At least this time, the food does not taste bad, it's just tasteless! The most important role that hemp plays in the whole process of detoxification is that it keeps the digestive tract extremely clean. This allows the toxins to be broken down an excreted in an extremely efficient manner, something that would not have been the case had it not been for hemp.

Kale: once a complete unknown in the world of health, kale is now widely considered to be one of the most important foods in the world as far as detoxification is concerned. Kale has one of the highest concentrations of antioxidants in the world, and they are also chocked full of phytochemicals as well. The antioxidants help to purify the blood and the phytochemicals obviously help the liver to break down the toxins in the blood stream so that they do not cause any damage in the body's digestive system. Kale is truly

174

a super food unlike any other!

Lemongrass: This herb is perhaps one of the oldest herbs that have ever been used for the purpose of cleansing the body. Used in the orient for at least hundreds of years, lemongrass has always been used for the specific purpose of cleansing organs of toxic chemicals. In fact, if you regularly consume lemongrass it will purge your entire digestive tract as well as your kidneys for you, meaning that your liver won't have to deal with any of this at all! Their cleaning of the digestive tract also makes it easier for the body to excrete toxic chemicals.

Lemons: Lemons are perhaps the poster boys of the entire detoxification movement, and for good reason too. They are instrumental for the liver to release its enzymes because the vitamins they contain are just so good for the liver. Lemons also induce the creation of alkaline chemicals in our digestive system, which is very important especially after we have eaten particularly spicy or rich foods that will be causing a lot of acidity. In general, lemons are perhaps the most important fruits that we can eat in our quest to detoxify our body and free ourselves of all foreign chemicals.

Olive oil: India got two, now Italy gets its second celebrated food in olive oil. It is one of the healthiest oils that you can use and is actually quite good at helping the liver to do its job and detoxify the body. It is low in fat and actually triggers a detoxification response in the liver, which is very important particularly when you are starting a detox diet. Even eating olive oil with your pizza or cooking your pasta in it can do your health a world of good, as olive oil is the healthiest oil that you can use.

Onions: Here we have a vegetable that is a stable for cuisines from around the world, and there is good reason for that. Not only are onions deliciously sharp, they are extremely healthy as well. The particular type of amino acids that onions contain provides a very specific benefit to the liver, which is that it detoxifies it. That's right, with all that detoxification the liver actually gets pretty toxic too! The onion helps it to become healthy and helps it to do its job as well, adding yet another vegetable into the category of super food.

Parsley: This is another example of a vegetable that is generally used as garnishing instead of being eaten outright that actually deserves to be eaten due to the immense health benefits that it provides. Chock full of vitamins A, B and even K, as well as large amounts of beta carotene, parsley is perhaps one of the most important vegetables you can eat while you are attempting to detox. Parsley also helps the body to reduce the amount of free radicals it has within it as well that helps to improve overall health and make the detoxification process a lot easier.

Pineapples: A delicious entry into this list at last! Pineapples aren't just one of the tastiest fruits around, they contain a little thing called bromelain which is absolutely essential to the health of your body and the detoxification process in general. Bromelain is a digestive enzyme that, of course, helps your body digest food. This means that it helps to cleanse the colon as well as the entire digestive tract that is an extremely important part of the detoxification process because it allows the body to flush the toxins that it has within it more efficiently.

Seaweed: Seaweed has recently come to be known as somewhat of a super food as well, with a lot of health experts beginning to promote it as being a great vegetable to eat. Indeed, it has been one of the most underrated vegetables for the longest time, especially considering the fact that it is able to bind itself to radioactive materials within our bodies and excrete them safely. This unique power of seaweed makes it an absolute must eat for us especially considering that we have absolutely no idea what it is that we are actually eating these days!

Sesame seeds: They are part of every good bun and add a savory goodness to them that we have come to take for granted, but sesame seeds are also extremely important because they are chock full of enzymes and antioxidants as well as important minerals, all of which are absolutely essential in our livers' struggle to dilute and break down the toxins that are present in our body. Sesame seeds also contain anti inflammatory agents which are very useful if you are suffering from swelling in any area of your body and don't want to use medicine.

Turmeric: this spice is essential because it aid both the liver as well as the digestive system. Its unique blend of nutrients is useful because it helps to optimize the liver's potential, allowing it to function at its maximum capacity. It also cleans out your digestive system, allowing your body to excrete the toxins it has within it in a more efficient manner. This double team of clean digestive system and optimum liver functionality is further boosted by the high antioxidant count that turmeric possesses. What all of this means is that turmeric should really be in your food!

Watercress: This vegetable is extremely important for your liver because it helps it to release the enzymes that it possesses within it and break down the toxic chemicals that have been built up within your body. It also possesses a lot of antioxidants that further help your body to detoxify itself.

Wheatgrass: This food is really important because of how much alkalinity it brings to your entire system. It works by reducing the acidity in your overall blood that is a very important way in which your body can detoxify itself, as toxins within your blood can make your blood acidic.

Chapter 14:

How Not to Detoxify Your Body – 10 Ways

While drinking water is a good detoxification measure, by itself it is not enough to get rid of the toxins you take n on a daily basis. There are plenty of other things that you need to be doing but there are also some things that you should be aware of. Going gung-ho into a detox plan will not work if you don't plan for it. Take not of these 10 ways on how NOT to detoxify your body.

1. Go Extreme

During a detox, you are going to be changing the way you eat, drink and behave but you do not need to go to extremes to accomplish this. Many people believe that a detox requires them to star themselves for a period of time and that it's going to hurt. This is not the case. The most successful detox plan will have you focusing on being calm and feeling well and healthy while feeding your body the nutrients it requires. Starving yourself will NOT achieve that.

2. Be Unprepared

Having the wrong attitude when it comes to detoxing your body is the fastest path to failure because you simply won't get the results you want. You must be prepared and you must know exactly what your plan is. Ask yourself these questions:

- How am I going to achieve this?
- How am I going to start?
- How long will I do this for?
- How will I get back to normal afterwards?

Of course, "normal" is going to be different so you need to work out what your new "normal" is going to be, Will you go back to how you were before or will you use this chance to change your ways? Ask yourself all of these questions and more before you start or you simply will not succeed.

3. Pick the wrong time to start

It is no good planning to start a detox plan when you are stressed out or at a busy time in your life. If you have a birthday coming up or the holidays are approaching, don't start a detox, wait until afterwards. Pick a time when there are likely to be few temptations and no distractions otherwise you simply will not stick to it and you will not reap any of the benefits. After holidays, after big parties or when you can take time off work and chill out are the best times.

4. Forget the water

It really doesn't matter which plan you choose to go with when you detox, there is one thing that is included in all of them – water. You may have to drink more water than you usually do but you must make the conscious effort to do so. Water is vital at any time but even more so when you are detoxing. This is because your organs are detoxing and need to get rid of the unhealthy impurities and toxins they are loaded with. They cannot do this if they do not have sufficient water to keep them hydrated. Drinking water regularly throughout the day helps to keep your internal workings running smoothly and to make sure you get enough water at a time when you may have to reduce your intake of food.

5. Ignoring the signals your body is sending

While you should always take note of your body, when you detox it is especially important. If, during your plan, you start to feel uncomfortable or in pain that is more than just hunger, do not continue pushing on and try to get past the pain. Speak to your doctor before you start a detox plan, as it may not be suitable for you or there may be contraindications that you need to be aware of. That way, you will be more certain about the pain, whether it is because of the detox or something else. You do need to be healthy to do a detox and if anything doesn't seem right, stop and, if necessary, seek medical advice

6. Rush in and rush out of a detox program

Both your mind and your body have to be ready for a detox so never rush in and just suddenly stop eating, or start of fruits and vegetables only for days and days on end. Your body needs to be eased in, to give it a chance to understand that things are changing. You must also prepare your mind for the changes ahead so it does not send your body into panic mode. At the other end of the plan, do not just rush out and go back to a normal diet. Again, you must ease your body back into it otherwise it will go into shock, especially if you start eating foods that you haven't eaten for several days.

7. Forget about your mind

So many people think that detoxing is just about the body and they forget about their minds. You can detox you mind just as well as you can your body. It's all about banishing negative thoughts, harmful thoughts and upsetting information and increasing the flow of positive information. Try doing a detox while watching the news when it's full of bad news and you will find that you will not be anywhere near as successful as you should be. You must detach yourself from all negative influences and relax.

8. Give in to the cravings

When you detox you are stopping the harmful flow of toxins into your body so it will do you no good whatsoever if, just after you start or halfway through, you give in to the inevitable cravings that will hit. It is only natural for your body to crave what you have always given it, especially when you suddenly take that substance away without warning. A good program will acknowledge your cravings and it will have a system for you to follow when those cravings hot. It will be a soup, a smoothie or a tea that can take the place of the food you crave.

Look at it this way – cravings are an excellent sign that the detox is working. Fight back against your body's screams and you will emerge triumphant and keep in mind that cravings only last a few minutes.

9. Keep switching between detox programs

You might think that the program you are eon is not working or that another plan looks far better, especially when you are halfway through it. What you must do, before you start on another plan, is finish the one you are on. You might not need to do another one if you let your current one run its course properly. Stopping and starting all the time will not get you the results you desire and you will not be any healthier.

Follow a program from start to finish and then leave it a while to assess the results before you jump straight in to another one. Giving up one plan for another is generally seen as a type of escape mechanism, one that allows you to get out of a program when the going gets a little too tough for you and you are unlikely to ever successfully complete a program.

10. Give it all up too soon

While it is important that you do not ignore the signals that your body is sending out, it is also important that you do not throw the towel in and give it all up when things start to get a little rough. More often than not, it is when you have got through a rough stage that the real detoxing and cleansing begins and you start to see the real positive effects of what you are doing. You must be able to work out what is considered normal and what isn't when it comes to the side effects of detoxing. Really and truthfully, to understand that, you need to be there throughout the entire process and that is the only way you are going to get the results that you are looking for. If necessary, join a couple of forums and get advice, support and help from those that have been there and successfully completed it.

These are the 10 biggest mistakes that are made by people starting out on a new detox program, especially in those that have never done one before. Avoiding these mistakes will make it more likely that you will succeed and you will reap the benefits from your detox program. Do not underestimate the ability that your body has in recovering from whatever you throw at it. The human body is remarkably resilient and stronger than you give it credit for. Al you are doing is giving it a helping hand, a respite from the hard work it does for you and it will respond positively when it knows that you are looking out for it. Keep that positive thought in your mind and success will be yours.

Conclusion

O nce again, thank you for downloading my book. I hope that I have been able to give you an oversight of what a detox is, how it works, and why we need to do it on a regular basis.

Anyone who is looking to kick start their weight loss, cleanse their systems so they feel better or simply give them back their youthful appearance will benefit from a detox cleanse. I must just reiterate that you should never carry out these plans long-term unless it is specified that you can. A proper diet detox can be done long term but those of you who are choosing the fruit or water detox must not go any further than 3-5 days without eating some form of proper food.

Please remember to seek medical advice if you are all unsure about whether a detox is right for you or if you have any condition that could make it dangerous. Your health is the most important thing and, although this is why we do a detox, doing one can worsen certain conditions.

CPSIA information can be obtained
at www.ICGtesting.com
Printed in the USA
BVHW070112090321
602012BV00003B/406